I0407130

Parent's Ear Infection Cookbook

● ● ● ●

Medical Recipes For Avoiding Surgery

Howard G. Smith M.D.

Cover design and illustration by Michael Jonathan.

Foreword

This book is dedicated to those professionals, patients, and parents who first taught me medicine and surgery and then helped me perfect the strategies contained in this book. I first thank the late Francis D. Moore, M.D., former Moseley Professor of Surgery at Harvard Medical School and former Surgeon-in-chief at Boston's Peter Bent Brigham Hospital, who introduced me to the science of surgery and taught me the skill of careful clinical observation. The late Harold F. Schuknecht, M.D., former Walter Augustus Lecompte Professor of Otology and Laryngology at Harvard and Chief of Otolaryngology at the Massachusetts Eye and Ear Infirmary, taught me how to medically as well as surgically correct ear disease and how to humanely as well as effectively care for the patient with those diseased ears. The late William W. Montgomery, M.D., the former Merriam Professor of Laryngology at Harvard, showed me that conscientious medical and surgical innovations make good therapy. The late Daniel Miller, M.D., former Clinical Professor of Otolaryngology at Harvard and Director of the Dana Farber Head and Neck Cancer Clinic, although a internationally renowned cancer surgeon, shared with me a wealth of good old fashioned medical otolaryngology "tips and tricks" as well as some clinical wisdom never taught to most of our younger physicians. Finally, I am most indebted to my mentor and colleague Gerald B. Healy, M.D., the former Healy Professor of Pediatric Otolaryngology at Harvard and the former Otolaryngologist-in-Chief at the Boston Children's Hospital, for teaching me the art and science of caring for children and their families and for encouraging my efforts to create innovative therapeutic approaches to children's ear, nose, and throat problems.

Over the past 35 years, I have had the privilege of caring for thousands of children and their families in Boston, Southern California, and Central Connecticut. The lessons that I have learned helping them hear, speak, and breathe better have led to the "recipes" in this book. I thank them all for adhering to the treatment plans and keeping their follow up appointments allowing me to determine the effectiveness of therapy. I am also indebted to their pediatricians for inviting me to collaborate with them in the care of their patients and families.

This book would have not been possible without the love and support of my parents Hilary and Lester Smith. They consistently encouraged me to direct my interests in science toward human biology and medicine. They also gifted me with both the intellect and the financial resources to pursue a career in medicine and surgery.

Special mega-thanks go to my partner in life and in medical practice, my wife Judy Goldstein Smith. A former speech-language pathologist, she has branched into medical office management, and she keeps our practice, Pediatric Ear, Nose & Throat Associates, humming and our patients pampered as well as satisfied. Her office design has created a healing environment second to none, and her love and understanding has given me the inspiration and freedom to continue perfecting these treatment techniques. I dedicate this book to her and to our children Michele, Greg, Michael, and David, for their love, support, and patience. May our first grandchild Lawson as well as thousands of children and grandchildren be the beneficiaries of these recipes.

Howard G. Smith, M.D.
West Hartford, Connecticut
August, 2011

Table of Contents

7 – Recipe for Air Humidification   147

Why do you need air humidification?
What is the ideal relative humidity?
How can you measure relative humidity?
When should you use a humidifier?
Which is the best type of humidifier?
Which brands of warm mist humidifiers are best?
What else can I do to achieve the healthiest air possible?

8 –Recipes for Allergies   153

What causes allergies?
How do environmental allergies cause ear disease?
How do you diagnose the existence of nasal and throat allergies?
When is a professional allergy evaluation worthwhile?
What are the recipes for preventing allergies?
What is the recipe for treating allergies?
Meet Lawson

9 – About Surgery   169

What types of surgery help middle ear problems?
What is "tube" surgery?
When should you consider this surgery for your child?
What are the benefits of this surgery?
What are the potential complication and risks of this surgery?
What follow up is necessary after this surgery?
Will my child require more than one set of "tubes?"
What are the details about the operative procedure to insert "tubes?"
What is "adenoid" surgery?
When should you consider this surgery for your child?
What are the benefits of this surgery?
What are the risks of this surgery?
What are the details of this surgery?

1 -- Introduction

You are likely reading this book because your child or grandchild has developed ear infections of the type that either recur or that will not clear. You are naturally concerned about the numbers and the amounts of medications, especially antibiotics, consumed. You are concerned that your child is often too ill to play or to attend day care, preschool or school. You are especially concerned about the ill effects of all this on your child's hearing and speech development. These issues are real and your concerns are appropriate.

My first piece of advice to you is to trust your intuition. Parents and grandparents know their infants and children best. If you have questions or worries, speak up and raise them with your child's doctors. One important goal of this book is to provide you with the information that will empower you as an advocate for your child.

Ear infections are common during infancy and childhood. They are the most common reasons for non-routine pediatrician visits. *Most* children will have fewer than three ear infections in a six-month period or four infections during a single calendar year. *Most* children will clear each infection quickly with the use of a single antibiotic at most. *Most* children will recover normal hearing within weeks following treatment of their ear infection. But your infant or child has proven to be different.

As a pediatric ear, nose, and throat specialist treating children and their ear infections for more than 30 years, I have learned what works as medical treatment and, most importantly, as prevention for ear infections. I have learned that most parents will do anything to help their kids get better once they understand the problem and its possible solutions. I have definitely learned that parents do not want their children to use excessive medication. Above all, parents wish to avoid surgery as part of the treatment for ear infections unless there are no other options. Despite that desire, artificial ventilation of the ears using tympanostomy tubes remains *the* most common surgical procedure performed on children in the United States today.

Our goal, yours and mine, is not to include your child in that statistic. We will succeed by preventing and managing your child's ear infections using the intelligent and timely application of medical therapy and medical therapy *alone*. We will succeed if you understand in common sense terms the causes of ear infections and how to help your child deftly sidestep them.

Good medical therapy is based on evidence from scientific studies. Unfortunately, the available data in the published literature does not offer us sufficient guidance for every aspect of treatment in every child. Like most clinicians, I use the observations and conclusions of published, controlled studies to modify and "fine tune" my own protocols which I have developed over years of clinical practice.

I urge you to read this material, follow its recommendations, and work with your own doctors who will provide the necessary clinical observations as outcome measures to determine the success of my recommended "recipes." Your own doctors will also provide the necessary prescription medications, including antibiotics, which are critical to the success of my regimens.

This is a cookbook with time-tested recipes for success. Each recipe includes necessary ingredients in the form of over-the-counter medications and prescription medications. Like most recipes, these will often work with alternate ingredients, and, like any good cook, you must discover which combinations of ingredients work best for your child and for you. Experiment, experiment, experiment! Keep notes on your calendars, PDAs, and iPhones about how much of which "ingredients" you used and what worked for your child.

In medicine, practice makes perfect, and I would love to hear from you about your own successful variations. Drop me a line at **earinfectioncookbook@gmail.com**. I will review your observations, try your suggestion myself, and likely add your recipe variations, your "better mousetraps," to future editions of my "cookbook."

Thank you for reading.

2 -- A Roadmap For Success: Understanding the Big Picture

Where is the site of common ear infections?
What is a middle ear infection?
What are the patterns of ear infections?
What causes ear infections to occur?
What causes ear infections to persist?
How to treat ear infections
How to prevent ear infections

Where is the site of common "ear infections?"

The most common ear infections during infancy and childhood are middle ear infections, in medical lingo termed *otitis media*. They occur in the so-called middle ear, the space located down the ear canal behind the eardrum. In contrast, another type of ear infection you have heard about, best known as "swimmers' ear" or otitis externa and more common in older children, adolescents, and adults, occurs in the ear canal itself or on the outer ear.

I already hear you asking, "Where are and what are all of these parts of the ear?" Well, it is important that you have a good understanding of how the ear is put together in order to understand how it gets infected. So let me first give you a mind's eye map of the ear. Also look at the illustrated simple "map" of the ear to get your bearings.

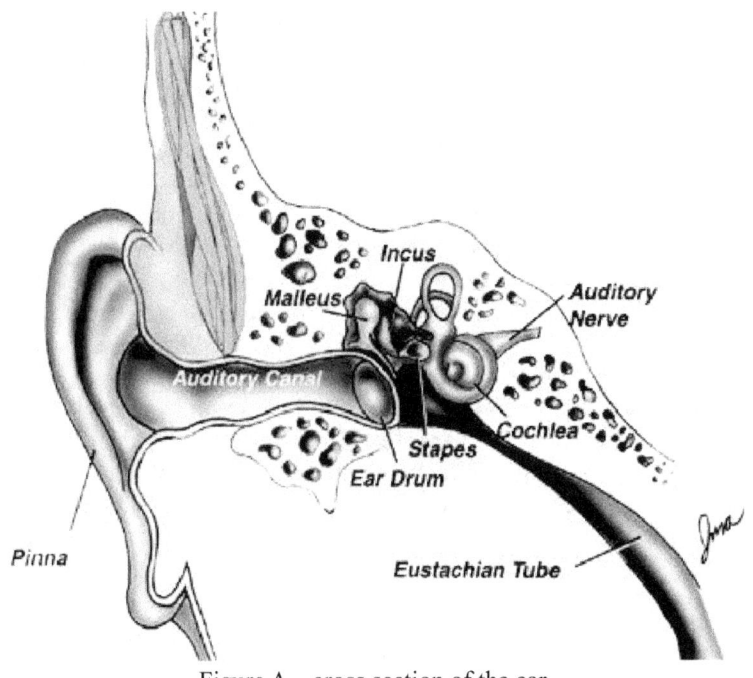

Figure A – cross section of the ear.
(Courtesy of the National Institutes of Health)

The part of the ear, which you see on the outside, is called the
auricle or *pinna.* It captures and funnels sound down the ear
canal toward the eardrum or *tympanic membrane.* Think of the
eardrum as a thin but watertight as well as airtight curtain
forming the outer wall of a tiny air-filled room in the side of the
head called the *middle ear space.* Sound waves hit the eardrum
and cause it to vibrate. Attached to the curtain and connecting it
to the far wall of the middle ear space is a chain of three tiny
bones or *ossicles.* When sounds shake the eardrum, this attached
chain freely rattles and shakes a little window on the wall
separating the middle ear from the inner ear. This so-called *oval
window* is a membrane sealing a porthole between the middle ear
space and the inner ear's labyrinth of fluid-filled circular

channels called the *cochlea*. When the eardrum and the attached ossicles rattle the oval window, the motion creates fluid waves in the cochlea that wash up against tiny hair-topped cells. These cells convert motion into electrical impulses which stream down the nerve of hearing to the brain and create the sense of sound.

Another part of the fluid-filled inner ear is the balance system. This ensemble of three semi-circular channels and a central lobby, the *vestibule*, connecting them responds to spinning or up-and-down head motions by creating fluid waves which wash up against sets of cells which also generate electrical impulses. These sensors in the semi-circular canals tell the brain the position of the head and the body. The balance system may be upset by the presence of ear infection or middle ear fluid, and a moderate proportion of children with middle ear problems become clumsy, experience falling episodes, or complain of dizziness.

The major focus of our efforts, yours and mine, is to keep your child's middle ear space filled with air and free of multiplying viruses and bacteria. This air-filled and infection-free middle ear status is necessary in order for your child to hear with normal sensitivity and full fidelity.

The middle ear space is closed except for a single ventilation route. The only way air or, for that matter, anything including agents of disease, can enter the middle ear chamber is through a narrow channel called the *eustachian tube*. This narrow passageway travels along the bottom of the skull and connects the front wall of the middle ear space to the back of the nose. The eustachian tube opens and closes as we breathe and swallow allowing air to flow from the back of the nose into the middle ear. When this air flows freely, it permits the pressure in the middle ear space to equal that in the ear canal and in your child's environment.

The air in the middle ear space must be consistently replaced since the oxygen within it is constantly being utilized by the living cells which compose the linings covering the middle ear walls, the ossicles, and the inside of the eardrum. If fresh air fails to travel up the eustachian tube into the middle ear and replace that which is used, the air pressure inside the middle ear "room" drops. Big trouble is just around the corner.

What is a middle ear infection?

A middle ear infection, better known as *otitis media*, is a process of rapid, uncontrolled turnover of bacteria or viruses within the middle ear space. The "germs" which trigger the infection may be forced up the eustachian tube by a sneeze, a cough, or nose blowing. Once they begin to multiply, they release some chemical substances and trigger the body to release others in defense, all of which cause the middle ear lining cells to become swollen and sometimes damaged. The swelling of the middle ear, eardrum, and eustachian tube linings then prevents fresh air from traveling up the eustachian tube and reaching the middle ear. When that occurs, air pressure within the middle ear space drops and a vacuum forms. This negative pressure draws more fluids, likely infected ones, up into the ear from the back of the nose. The negative pressure itself as well as tissue damage resulting from bacterial and viral activity also causes fluid to form in the normally air-filled middle ear space. This fluid, called a *middle ear effusion*, makes an ideal culture medium for additional bacterial growth. Think of a middle ear infection, an otitis media, as a downward spiral. Infection causes tissue swelling, eustachian tube blockage, a drop in middle ear pressure, fluid formation, and more infection. And so it goes . . . .

Once the infection is rolling, your child may develop any number of possible symptoms and signs or none at all. Commonly, ongoing otitis media causes ear pain that may be worse when lying down, general irritability, wakefulness, loss of appetite, temporary hearing diminution, and balance problems.

As your child's immune system fights the infection and kills off the viruses and bacteria, the middle ear and eustachian tube lining swelling gradually diminishes allowing air to once again enter the middle ear space. As this occurs, the middle ear fluid dries up and the ear returns to its normal, healthy state.

On the other hand, in the worst-case scenario, the body may not be able to stop the growth of the viruses and bacteria. Their continued proliferation leads to tremendous swelling and the build-up of pressure in the middle ear space and the development of a "pop off valve," a perforation, in the eardrum. The latter usually heals quickly, but its occurrence signals a severe ear infection.

Sometimes, unrelieved middle ear pressure may drive back flow of infected fluid back into the mastoid chamber, an air-filled cavity located behind the middle ear space, thus creating a nasty infection called acute *mastoiditis*. The pus may also be pushed out of the mastoid cavity proper into the adjacent fluid-filled space around the brain causing *meningitis*. The two m's, mastoiditis and meningitis, are two complications of middle ear disease which are most feared. Since the introduction of antibiotic treatment for otitis media, these complications have been all but eliminated. In fact, their prevention is the chief reason for treating ear infections with antibiotics at all.

During ear infections and the recovery periods that follow them, your child's hearing will be diminished. The hearing loss is caused by the poor conduction of sound from the surface of the eardrum to the inner ear. The negative pressure in the middle ear and fluid within the middle ear space both prevent the eardrum from moving properly. Hearing impairment also occurs due to tissue swelling of the eardrum and the linings around the chain of bones conducting the vibrations. During these times, the hearing is muffled. Usually, both the volume level of sound a child hears and the fidelity of the sound are reduced. This type of hearing deterioration interferes with efficient speech-language development. The good news is that the hearing loss is temporary. One caveat: the longer it takes for your child's ear tissues to return to normal, the longer your child will experience suboptimal hearing, both in terms of loudness and fidelity and clarity.

What are the patterns of ear infections?

Acute and recurrent is the most common pattern of troublesome ear infection in infants. Typically, this pattern is characterized by the occurrence of acute ear infections in one or both ears in association with upper respiratory infections such as run of the mill "colds." Each infection resolves quickly and completely after initiation of therapy. **Acute and persistent** infections are symptomatic episodes that require multiple antibiotics for effective treatment or fail to respond to a succession of ever stronger and more competent antibiotics. **Subacute and persistent** ear infections are associated with milder inflammatory changes of the eardrum and middle ear tissues compared with acute infections, and many are asymptomatic or only mildly symptomatic infections. These bouts, despite their low intensity, continue despite the use of strong antibiotic treatments. **Chronic and recurrent** ear infection bouts are repetitive episodes during which middle ear fluid and hearing loss predominate in contrast to acutely painful inflammation and infection. For children with **chronic and persistent** ear infections, middle ear inflammation, middle ear fluid and hearing losses persist over many weeks and months without the occurrence of an acute ear infection.

What causes acute middle ear infections to occur?

The answer to this question is simple: AN INFECTION IN THE NOSE AND UPPER THROAT. Since the only way in and out of the middle ear is through the eustachian tube channel, all contamination of the middle ear is caused by germs passing from the back of the nose and upper throat, technically called the *nasopharynx*, into the middle ear space.

The most common culprit is the common cold, a viral infection of the nasal linings. The virus is usually picked up on the hands, passed from hand to mouth, mouth to mid-throat, mid-throat to upper throat, upper throat to the back of the nose, and from the back of the nose up through the eustachian tube into the middle ear and forward through the nasal cavities into the sinuses. Nose blowing, sneezing, and coughing will all accelerate viral passage into the middle ear and nose. Once the viruses set up housekeeping in either the middle ear space or within the nasal or sinus cavities, the body's immune system begins to quickly eliminate them, but the secondary tissue swelling in these zones may then permit bacteria, which are also present, to multiply and create a secondary infection.

Sometimes, a bacterial middle ear infection may develop without a preexisting viral infection of the nasal linings if nasal bacteria are "blown" up into the middle ear. This may occur during the latter phases of "colds" or bronchial infections. This problem may be avoided with proper precautions, and I will discuss in detail how to manage "colds" in a later chapter.

Another common scenario that may trigger a middle ear infection is the development of eustachian tube swelling at its nasal end. This swelling is caused by one or more of the following problems: post-nasal drainage from nasal and sinus infections; nasal allergic reactions such as the seasonal spring "rose fever," the autumn "hay fever." or year round allergies;

physical irritation of the nasal and throat linings by passive smoke from sources such as cigarettes, cigars, fireplaces, and wood-burning stoves; or the "backwash" of irritating liquids such as milk, formula, juice, and stomach acid, so-called *reflux,* into the upper throat. My recipes also cover solutions to these problems.

Sometimes, otitis media occurs, or I should say recurs, because the middle ear fluid and tissue reaction from a previous bout have not completely resolved. Bacteria and other infectious organisms may persist in a thin film called a *biofilm*, which then coats the linings of the middle ear spaces and eustachian tubes. A slight and temporary drop in a child's immune strength is then all that is needed for these germs to reactivate and trigger an ear infection.

What causes ear infections to persist?

A middle ear infection persists for two reasons. ONE: your child's body cannot eliminate the viruses or bacteria that caused it. TWO: the middle ear lining swelling fails to resolve due to the inability of the eustachian tube to open and readmit a sufficient quantity of air.

It is rare that a pure viral infection will persist in the middle ear, since your child's immune system makes such a vigorous reaction to it. More commonly, a bacterial infection, which follows the viral infection, persists due to the presence of one or more bacteria that are resistant to the antibiotic used. Unfortunately, over the past ten years, bacteria commonly found in the ears, noses, and throats of infants and children have become increasingly resistant to many frequently prescribed antibiotics. These very resistant bacteria are commonly found in children attending day care and pre-school, and, as a result, such children are more prone to infections, which resist all but the stronger antibiotics.

Bacteria have become more resistant to antibiotics due to the overuse of these medications, particularly in low doses for longer periods of time. In order to stop this process and to avoid arriving at a time when some if not many bacteria will be resistant to all antibiotics, we must become "smarter" about our use these "miracle drugs." We must use them more selectively and employ treatment strategies that kill the bacteria rather than select out resistant strains.

Reopening the middle ear to a "breath of fresh air" may be quite challenging, and failure to do so with medical therapy alone is the most common reason for resorting to surgery. The only natural route for that "fresh air" to enter the ear is through the eustachian tube ventilation ports at the back of your child's nose. If that nose is running faster than Niagara Falls and smells like a toxic waste dump, you won't be surprised to hear that the nasal entrances to your child's eustachian tubes will remain blocked to air passage or will admit contaminated material into the middle ear. If the eustachian tubes do open and attempt to let air in, the swollen and contaminated middle ear linings tend to remain that way as swelling begets infection and infection leads to swelling. Turning the tide may be like dredging the Everglades.

How to treat ear infections.

Ear infections resolve when your child's immune system eliminates the viruses and, with the help of antibiotics, the bacteria which cause them and when air reenters your child's middle ear spaces to help thin their linings. All measures which enhance the function of your child's immune system help this process including: good nutrition, sufficient sleep, and avoidance of other drains on immune system energy. You help your child's immune system work in high gear by arranging for your child to avoid other children who are actively sick and by steering your child clear of nasal and throat irritants such as smoke, chemicals, and, if your child is sensitive, airborne allergens such as pollens, dust, and mold.

The use of antibiotics helps your child's immune system prevent bacterial growth, but antibiotics are not a panacea. To fight increasingly more resistant bacteria, we continue to develop stronger and stronger antibiotics and better recipes for combining them in order to kill even the most devious bacteria. This is a moving target, however, and the medications, which work during this month or this year, may be relatively ineffective in the future.

The most important measures involve re-ventilating the middle ear spaces by driving air up from the nose into the ear through the eustachian tubes. These include eliminating nasal infections and nasal allergic reactions along with the nasal lining swelling which accompanies them. We accomplish this with the use of nasal cleansing and decongestion regimens and with the use of anti-allergic and anti-inflammatory medications.

You have undoubtedly read that pediatricians, family physicians, and ear, nose and throat specialists are now recommending that we all attempt to minimize the use of antibiotic therapy. The latest recommendations suggest taking a wait-and-see (**WAS**) attitude toward the treatment of acute ear infections delaying the start of antibiotics for several days while treating any symptoms such as pain and fever with over-the-counter drugs such as the aspirin substitutes *Tylenol*™, *Advil*™, or *Motrin*™. If a child's symptoms persist or escalate in the absence of antibiotic therapy, it is then begun on a delayed basis.

This **WAS** strategy is suggested for infants above the age of 6 months and children with a normal number and severity of ear infections. If you are reading this book, chances are excellent that your child does not fall into this category. For infants and children with increased natural tendencies to develop ear infections, a delay initiating appropriate antibiotic therapy may permit their infections to advance more rapidly creating tissue changes with will serve to prolong their recovery from the infection and which will make subsequent infections more probable.

How to prevent middle ear infections.

Most ear infections are triggered by "colds" and other upper respiratory infections such as sore throats and bronchitis. Preventing as many of these as possible will prevent the majority of middle ear infections. Do this by keeping your child away from other children who have "colds," and thereby preventing transmission of "colds" from child to child. Much has been written in parents' magazines about how to do this, but *my* list is headed by preventive measures including hand washing, cleaning of shared toys, avoiding pacifier use, humidification, and nasal cleansing. We will discuss much more about all of this later.

How many ear infections are too many?

Since all children have ear infections, when should you as a parent become concerned? The following scenarios should trigger concern and suggest the need for more intense preventive therapy and treatment including the care of a specialist:
• 4 or more acute middle ear infections in a 12-month period;
• 3 or more acute middle ear infections in a 6-month period;
• 2 or more acute middle ear infections associated with a perforation;
• 1 acute middle ear infection per month for more than 3 months;
• 1 acute middle ear infection that persists for longer than 3 to 4 weeks, especially if the child is very irritable, wakeful, feverish and clearly ill;
• Fluid observed in both ears for more than two months if your child seems to be experiencing hearing and/or speech difficulties;

• Fluid observed in both ears for more than three months even if your child seems to be hearing appropriately;
• Fluid observed in one ear for more than three months if your child seems to be experiencing hearing and/or speech difficulties.

If any of these situations arise in your child, ask for a conference with your child's pediatrician. Indicate your concerns, and ask the pediatrician to make a list of your child's ear infections, the circumstances in which they arose, and their treatment. This objective look at your child's clinical history, the "rap sheet" of otitis media, often suggests a pattern and an approach to treatment.

Once you and your pediatrician review your child's ear infection history, you should be able to jointly arrive at a strategy for managing this problem going forward. The recipes in this book provide a framework for maximal medical management. Your pediatrician may wish to implement them or variations on them directly. More likely, your pediatrician will suggest that you take your child to an ear, nose, and throat specialist for a consultation. Following that visit, your pediatrician will work closely with that specialist to provide an effective treatment program.

Remember that referral to a specialist should not automatically guarantee a trip to the operating room. Otolaryngologists are in the best position to help your pediatrician craft treatment programs and to provide serial clinical monitoring to assess the success or failure of such programs. If your pediatrician tells you that the specialist referral is merely for a preoperative examination, ask for an explanation. If, after reading this book and other literature available to you, that explanation is unsatisfying, request a referral to a specialist who will fairly and evenhandedly review your child's history, his or her current clinical status, and recommend comprehensive medical management before resorting to surgery. You want a specialist who will not merely rubber-stamp another physician's opinion but one who will apply creative problem-solving and suggest a treatment plan which tilts the benefit-risk "see-saw" in your child's favor.

3 -- Recipes for Recurring Acute Otitis Media

Meet Mikey

To understand the issues surrounding recurrent otitis media, let's look at a typical infant suffering from this type of ear disease. Let me introduce you to Mikey, a sweet and mellow little fellow, whom I first met at 15 months of age. He is the first child of two committed and doting first time parents, George and Lori. George is a software engineer and Lori teaches fourth grade. She took maternity leave for the remainder of the school year following his birth, and she was nursing him. Then, in late

August, at 5 months of age, Mikey began attending the KiddieCare day care center as Lori headed back to her classroom. By late September, he experienced his first "cold." Three days after his nose began to run, his lovely disposition disappeared and he began to cry and whine incessantly, refuse his bottle, shriek when positioned on his back for diaper changes, refuse to fall asleep, and awaken repeatedly. Mom and dad carted him off to see Dr. Brown, his pediatrician, who diagnosed his first set of ear infections.

Mikey cleared quickly on one course of the antibiotic *amoxicillin*, and, although he experienced one minor "cold," he remained free of ear infections for two months. Then just after Thanksgiving, he developed another "cold" followed rapidly by a left-sided ear infection. At his two-week follow up visit, the course of amoxicillin had helped to erase the inflammation in his left eardrum, but he did have a fluid collection in his middle ear space. This cleared by the time he came in for his 9-month well-child exam.

His "Happy New Year" celebration was anything but happy. Instead of watching the Big Apple's crystal ball drop while basking in the flickering light of the family wood-burning stove, he and his folks spent the night at the Children's Hospital emergency room (ER) for evaluation and treatment of fever and irritability. The ER docs ruled out meningitis, but they diagnosed Mikey with bilateral ear infections. This third episode of infection was treated with a stronger antibiotic, cefdinir or *Omnicef.* The infection cleared quickly, but diminishing amounts of fluid were seen in each ear for weeks after. What then followed was a run of three additional ear infections occurring 3 to 4 weeks apart, each with a "cold," and many requiring more than one antibiotic to control.

His last ear infection was so fierce that he developed a perforated left eardrum. Treatment for this monster otitis media event included amoxicillin 600 mg + potassium clavulanate, better known as *Augmentin ES* (Extra Strength) and *ofloxacin* (*Floxin*) eardrops, a topical antibiotic drop. After this sixth infection resolved in early April, Dr. Brown recommended that Mikey remain on a two-month low dose course of the amoxicillin. This regimen worked like a charm for about 6 weeks. Then, in late May, his entire day care was attacked by "cold-zilla." Despite the "protective" course of amoxicillin, he developed a seventh episode of otitis media in each ear and a nasty sinus infection. By the time I first met him as a patient in mid-June, these infections had survived courses of broad-spectrum antibiotics including azithromycin or Zithromax, cefuroxime axetil or *Ceftin*, and *Augmentin ES*, which he was just finishing.

Mikey's case illustrates common features of recurring otitis media during infancy. As I review it with you, I will give you a "cooking demonstration." You will peek in on his visits with me, and I will review the recipes that I used to successfully stop his and many other children's cycles of recurrent otitis media.

Mikey's First Visit

By the time of his first visit with me in mid-June, Mikey had just finished his course of *Augmentin ES* as treatment for his seventh otitis media and a sinus infection. When I first met his parents, George and Lori, they were understandably upset and frightened. Every new otitis media brought sleepless nights and crabby days. Even his customary bottle before bed failed to completely calm him, and he was drinking another in the middle of the night. He was so irritable that he craved his pacifier constantly.

Though he seemed to hear well enough and loved listening to his bedtime stories, his vocabulary was no longer growing. Babbling constantly in the months leading up to his first birthday, he had 3 words by the time of his birthday celebration and 8 words the following month. His word acquisition was now stalled, and the words he did use were no longer clearly recognizable.

His folks told me that each of them had ear infections as infants and toddlers. Dad had tubes inserted, and mom eventually underwent tonsillectomy and adenoidectomy. Mom and dad both tend to experience seasonal congestion but neither of them carries an official diagnosis of allergic rhinitis.

After reviewing Mikey's history with his parents and after combing through his pediatrician's records, my exam began. As I examined Mikey's ears with a handheld ear microscope, I found that his eardrums were thickened but not inflamed. This indicated that the antibiotics had done their jobs and helped to eliminate the infection. His middle ear spaces appeared filled with air. My sonar ear probe, the instrument known as a *tympanometer*, confirmed that air was present in Mikey's middle ear spaces but that the air pressure in each ear was lower than desirable. This situation occurs because the thickened linings of his eustachian tubes and middle ear spaces prevent the amount of air necessary to maintain normal middle ear pressures from entering the middle ear with each swallow or yawn. After any ear infection and particularly after a run of them, it takes time for the lining thickening to disappear. While the linings remain thickened, Mikey's chances of redeveloping another ear infection remain elevated.

My examination of Mikey's nasal cavities provided a clue to his problem. His nasal linings were moderately thickened and he had substantial amounts of mucus within each nasal cavity, particularly at the back of each nasal cavity. His mouth and throat exam were normal, except that he was teething.

Mikey's history and clinical presentation at exam is fairly typical of infants with recurrent otitis media. First of all, little boys in general and children whose parents have a history of otitis media are more likely to develop their own problem with ear infections. Most infants are protected from usual childhood infections for their first six months of life by maternal antibodies transferred through the placenta during the gestational period. Breast-feeding definitely helps accentuate this natural immunity by providing additional maternal antibodies through breast milk. In many cases such as Mikey's, breast-feeding may improve the situation but it does not prevent recurrent ear infections.

A cascade of events has led to Mikey's current ear infection issues. His exposure in day care has driven a series of upper respiratory infections. These, in turn, triggered the ear infections. Successive bouts of otitis media then led to chronic swelling of the eardrum, middle ear linings, and eustachian tube linings. The swelling makes it difficult for air to reach his middle ear spaces and drive their return to normal after an infection has resolved. This same pattern has also occurred in Mikey's nasal cavities and sinuses.

The VIP Program for Recurrent Otitis Media

My master recipe for Mikey's woes is the **VIP** program, well titled since your children and my patients are VIPs. This acronym stands for **Ventilation** and **Infection Prevention.**

This **VIP** recipe is two individual but interrelated recipes, one for **ventilation** and the other for **infection prevention**. The rationale behind this blend of recipes is the fact that, for the ears, as well as for the nasal cavities and the sinuses, lining swelling leads to infection and infection leads to lining swelling. Since ear infections produce tissue swelling and that swelling, in turn, leads to the recurrence and persistence of infection and middle ear fluid, a major blast of "fresh air" is necessary to clean the swamp!

VENTILATION
The goal of my ventilation recipe is to direct air into Mikey's middle ear spaces, nasal passages, and sinus cavities. The air allows his linings in both the ears and nose to return to normal and, in so doing, makes it less likely for future infections to

occur and more likely for high fidelity sound transmissions to occur.

Ventilation occurs by **cleansing** and **decongesting** the nasal linings. I am always concerned about the state of a child's nasal linings, even if sinusitis has not been an issue, because the nasal passages are the conduits for air into the ear and they may be a repository for infection. The only natural air vent for the middle ear space is the eustachian tube, located at the back of each nasal cavity.

CLEANSING

My cleansing routine begins with an emphasis on maintaining clean and moist linings within the nose, throat, and, of most importance, within the eustachian tubes and middle ear spaces. It consists of saline mist irrigations for the nose and humidification as well as cleansing of the air your child breathes.

Saline mist irrigation:

The linings of our throat, noses, eustachian tubes and ears are so called *mucous membranes*, and they must remain moist in order for them to function normally. Think of these mucous membrane linings as miniature conveyor belts with a blanket of mobile mucus lying on a layer of cells with tiny moving hairs on top of them called *cilia*. It is these cilia that "motorize" the mucus and allow it to perform its natural cleansing process. Without this cleansing and emptying process, bacteria, molds, virus-laden mucus, and allergens will stall, accumulate, and foster localized infection. Dryness also creates direct damage to the ciliated membranes in the same way as it does to the skin. This damage allows germs to enter the body and trigger infection.

To provide this necessary moisturization, I recommend instillation of over-the-counter saline sprays, available as *Simply Saline, Ocean, or Little Noses Saline* mist in an aerosol sprayer. I prefer the use of either the aerosol or manual pump packaging as one-way valves in these prevent the back flow of nasal mucus from the tip back into the container, thus avoiding contamination of the remainder of the saline. Most squeeze bottles do not have one-way valves in the spray tip. The aerosol packaging method is also advantageous since the solution is delivered from a pressurized, sealed container, eliminating the need for squeezing the bottle and the need for preservatives. These chemical preservatives can irritate the sensitive linings of infants and children. The aerosol packing also includes a removable tip, which permits the nozzle to be cleaned after use. I recommend warming the saline can or bottle to body temperature by keeping the container in a parental shirt pocket prior to use.

Spray two sprays in each nostril three times a day, and use even more often during "colds." Allow the mist to cover the intranasal linings, mix with mucus, and then wend its way to the back of the nose. Do not suction the saline back out the front of the nose with the little bulb syringe that was a part of your newborn kit. This maneuver may pull contaminated material from the back of the nasal cavity and the adenoidal mass into the "cleaner" environment of the middle and anterior nasal cavity.

I instructed Mikey's parents to instill the saline mist in the morning before he departed for day care, when he returned from day care, and just before he went to sleep at night. Mikey, like most infants, did not initially "love" the nasal sprays. After the successive saline spraying led to healthier nasal linings, Mikey instinctively realized that his nose was feeling better as the result of the saline, and he began to look for it. Of course, he continued to look for the reward as well.

The regular use of saline mist irrigation "flushes" away infecting organisms entering the back of the nose and thereby reduces the incidence of viral "colds," allergic nasal inflammation, and secondary bacterial infections of the ears, nasal cavities, and sinuses. The saline also restores a normal consistency to nasal mucus that has "sludged" as the result of your child breathing dry air. Nasal and throat mucus must be thin enough to move in the proper direction in order to maintain clean nasal cavities, eustachian tube entrances, and nasal sinuses. The saline also flushes away overabundant mucus, and, in so doing, acts as a decongestant.

Humidification:
Nasal and throat linings swell more readily when they are dry. Consistent use of a humidifier to maintain the relative humidity in your child's room between 40 to 45% is critical in order to maintain sufficiently moist and healthy linings in the nose, throat, eustachian tubes, and, most importantly, in the middle ear. I recommend that you keep an inexpensive **humidity gauge**, a *hygrometer*, in your child's room. Such gauges are available at hardware stores, with mechanical versions priced under $10 and electronic versions in the $10 to $30 range.

Once you know the humidity level in your child's room, you will likely need to increase it, particularly during the cooler seasons when your home furnace is blazing. For this task, I recommend the use of a **warm mist humidifier** such as a model manufactured by Honeywell or Vicks. Currently, most of the warm mist humidifiers are made by the same company, Kaz. Look for a model with a 2 or more gallon capacity, a humidistat which controls the vapor production to prevent the room from becoming too humid, and, ideally, a safety fan to mix the pure water vapor with room air. Many of the newer models lack a fan, and, if you purchase one of those, I suggest that you purchase an external safety fan with soft rubber blades. Position it to blow room air over the hot air outlet of the humidifier. This effectively mixes the hot vapors from the humidifier with the cooler room air and circulates the humidified air around the room.

Use the humidity gauge to set the humidifier to the desired level by tuning the humidifier on and turning its humidistat all the way up to initially maximize vapor production. Dial back the humidistat to stop the vapor production once the humidity gauge indicates that the relative humidity in the room is between 40 and 45 percent.

Mikey's folks told me that they had several old humidifiers around the house. One was a cold mist model and the other was an ultrasound model. I told them to throw both out in the garbage after cutting off the cords so that an unsuspecting garbage can scavenger with a child would not be tempted to use them. To find out why these types of humidifiers are downright dangerous, see the chapter *A Recipe for Air Humidification*.

Air cleansing:
Keep your child away from dirty air. Do not smoke in the house or, preferably, at all. Cigarette, cigar, and pipe smoke sticks to everything, and it easily enters your home and your child's respiratory system on your clothes. Clean the rooms in your home often and try to keep your child out of rooms where you are dusting, vacuuming, woodworking, or using strong and smelly solvents. Avoid the use of wood-burning stoves or fireplaces. If your home seems unusually dusty, consider purchasing an air cleaner. Consult consumer information sources such as reviews on the internet via Google searches for reviews of current models.

Fortunately, neither of Mikey's parents smoke, but the family does have a wood-burning stove. They discontinued its use.

Prevent stomach reflux:
We have long known that milk or other foods easily pass up from the mouth and upper throat into the back of the nose when infants and toddlers feed lying down. For this reason, pediatricians and ear, nose, and throat specialists have long recommended feeding infants and toddlers in the upright position. Recent research now also indicates that food recently ingested and retained in the stomach as well as the stomach acid it produces often comes back up into the upper airway and throat if an infant or toddler lies down to sleep or nap too soon after eating. These irritating fluids may rise high enough to bathe the back of the nose, the eustachian tube inlets, and the adenoids. This so-called *extra esophageal reflux* produces nasal

congestion, inflammation of the adenoids, eustachian tube dysfunction, and, ultimately, the formation of middle ear fluid.

Since the stomach may require as long as 90 minutes to empty following a meal, avoid feeding your child just before bedtime or a nap. Try to compartmentalize feeding to other parts of the day. If you want to give a "security nightcap," give water in the bottle or cup. If you must feed just before bed or nap, maintain your child in an upright position as sleep comes on by placing your infant or toddler in a swing or car seat. After 60 to 90 minutes, transfer the child to the crib. It is also sometimes helpful to elevate the head of the crib or bed using a pillow or two *under* the mattress or by using blocks under the legs at the head of the crib.

Some children have other evidence of gastroesophageal reflux disease and extra-esophageal reflux disease. Footprints of these problems include not only the obvious regurgitation of food, but also more subtle symptoms such as nighttime and morning cough, throat pain, and hoarseness. When such symptoms coexist with ear infection problems, diagnostic efforts should be made to verify the occurrence of reflux. Once confirmed, reflux should be initially managed with acid suppression therapy using agents such as *ranitidine* (*Zantac)* or *lansoprazole* (*Prevacid)*.

Mikey's parents will move his bedtime bottle back several hours and give him a cup of water just before bed or nap time. They have a wind up swing and will use it or use his car seat if necessary. He has no symptoms to suggest significant gastroesophageal reflux disease or extra-esophageal reflux disease.

Consider allergies:
Many infants and toddlers begin to show evidence of seasonal or year-round allergies as they grow. Keep your index of suspicion high while looking for nasal, throat, airway, or eye irritation as the result of exposures at home and out of doors. Look for reactions when you are dusting and cleaning the house, exposing

your child to cats and dogs, or spending time out of doors near flowers or freshly cut grass. This risk of allergy in your child is significantly higher if one or if both parents have or had allergies themselves.

If your child only experiences characteristic nasal congestion and nasal drainage at certain times of the year, in certain environments, or after very specific exposures, the diagnosis is nearly made. A formal allergy evaluation may be useful, but it is not mandatory since your pediatrician or ear, nose, and throat specialist will suggest and prescribe a treatment program. On the other hand, if there is evidence of allergic reactions for more than 4 months of the year, ask your pediatrician or specialist about an allergy consultation. Read more about my treatment for allergies in the chapter *Recipes for Allergies*.

Mikey's parents both have a history of seasonal allergies, and that fact significantly increases his chances of developing allergies. They have not noticed any tendency for him to have chronic nasal congestion or symptoms of post-nasal drainage at those times of the year when they are affected. He makes no reactions to his grandmother's dog and cat. They will continue to observe him closely.

DECONGESTION

The goal of my decongestion recipe is to maintain a child's nasal and throat linings in their normal, non-swollen state. By using the steps listed for the cleansing recipe just above, you are already beginning to decongest your child. But . . . there is much more that you can do.

My decongestion recipe, which I nickname the **SADDS** (pronounced 'sads') program, is a step regimen that instructs parents to use a number of various decongesting agents. I mention the agents in the order of suggested addition. I recommend that parents use as few or as many of these ingredients as necessary knowing that all ingredients may be used individually or in combination with each other. The only ingredient that I feel should always be in use is the saline mist irrigation. Otherwise, I ask that parents feel free to vary the recipe to improve effectiveness and acceptance.

Decode the **SADDS** acronym as follows:

S:	**saline mist irrigation**
A:	**oral anti-inflammatory agent**
D:	**oral decongestant**
D:	**topical decongestant**
S:	**topical steroid nasal spray**

Let's look at the individual components of the **SADDS** program. They are:

Saline mist irrigation:

Once again, our old friend saline comes to the rescue. If you define decongestion as the elimination of nasal obstructive tendencies, the simplest way to achieve that goal is to flush away accumulating mucus with saline mist nasal irrigation. This is the first and most basic step in my decongestion program. The saline may be instilled as often as necessary during the day. For most infants and children with ear, nose, and throat infection issues, I recommend at least 2 sprays in each nostril at least 3 times a day, every day. For those with active "colds" or upper respiratory infections, I suggest that parents increase the frequency of saline administration. I recommend the same 2 sprays in each nostril but they should be instilled every 2 to 3 hours during the time a child is awake.

Oral anti-inflammatory agents:

For more vigorous treatment of nasal symptoms, usually necessary during "colds" and nasal allergy attacks, you must add specific medications to the saline mist nasal irrigations. In most children excepting younger infants under 6 months, the first medications that I recommend using are the anti-inflammatory agents.

The most useful and safe anti-inflammatory agents are members of a class known as non-steroidal anti-inflammatory drugs, abbreviated as **NSAIDs**. Included in this family are the widely-used medications *ibuprofen* (*Motrin*, *Advil* or the generic equivalents) and *naproxen* (*Aleve*). Another NSAID is *aspirin*, but **ASPIRIN SHOULD NEVER BE USED IN CHILDREN** due to its association with a deadly, necrotizing form of liver inflammation known as Reye's Syndrome. NSAIDs reduce inflammation by counteracting the cyclooxygenase (COX) enzyme which help to synthesize prostaglandins, important creators of tissue swelling and increased lining secretions.

You likely already use these drugs after athletic injuries such as ankle sprains. In addition to alleviating pain, they stop swelling of the injured tissues and the accumulation of fluid between cells. Think of "colds" and other forms of rhinitis as a "sprained nose," and using the NSAIDS will reduce nasal congestion, anterior and post-nasal drainage, as well as nasal and throat lining sensitivity leading to less sneezing and coughing. NSAIDS also help control the fever associated with viral infections.

These "miracle" drugs, however are imperfect "miracles." They, like aspirin, can irritate stomach linings, thin the blood, and, in a select number of individuals, exacerbate asthma. For this reason, they must be used carefully, taken on a full stomach, and, in those with gastrointestinal issues, asthma, bleeding tendencies, or upcoming/recent surgery, only used with the advice and consent of your child's pediatrician.

Oral decongestants:
The anti-inflammatory medications generally function well as decongestants, and they reduce the lining swelling within the nasal cavities and sinuses as well as reduce nasal secretions and post-nasal drainage. However, at the mid-portion of the viral nasal infection, they often need help. This help comes in the form of oral and topical decongestants. These medications perform their function by "squeezing" blood vessels in nasal

tissues and elsewhere thereby preventing the engorgement of nasal linings and their production of mucus secretions in response to the viral infection. The oral decongestants may be used in infants over 6 months of age and in children and adolescents of any age. Since they compress all blood vessels, they should be only used with great caution in those with heart or vascular disease.

My favorite oral decongestant is *Sudafed,* the brand name for over-the-counter drugs containing the chemical *pseudoephedrine.* This drug is available in liquid form as *Sudafed Children's Decongestant Liquid,* in short-acting tablet form, and in extended release tablet form. Typically begin using the decongestant by using one dose before bedtime, and that may be the only dose necessary. The reason decongestants have the most dramatic effect on your child at night is because they are replacing the missing natural adrenalin which is present during the day. Because the adrenalin is missing at night, the nasal, sinus, and eustachian tube linings swell and produce more secretions. This phenomenon explains why most of us awaken with nasal "stuffiness" in the morning and experience post-nasal drainage at night. If one dose of the decongestant before bedtime is not sufficient to keep your child's nasal linings open, add an additional dose in the middle of the night. Oral decongestants may be given up to 4 times a day or every 4 to 6 hours.

For older children and adolescents who are able to swallow tablets, caplets, or capsules, *Sudafed* and its generic equivalents are available in conventional tablets and extended release forms. The conventional tablets are dosed every 4 to 6 hours. The extended release tablets and capsules will last 8 to 12 rather than 4 hours, and allow effective dosing through the night and during the school day. By the way, many younger children who are unable to swallow a pill will easily swallow a "glob" of peanut butter or marshmallow fluff with a pill embedded in its middle.

Infants and toddlers should use Children's *Sudafed*. How much should you use? The package will almost always say, "For children under the age of 6, ask your doctor." OK, you have, and I will share with you the doctors' formula for determining the dosage for your children in the **Appendix**.

If the use of Sudafed keeps your child up at night, you may also give a dose of *Benadryl* along with the *Sudafed*. This medication will neutralize most of the stimulation provided by the *Sudafed*, and it will also help your child sleep better. The unfortunate side effect is that it dries all linings. One potential negative of using antihistamine-containing compounds is the possibility that they may thicken middle ear fluid. A number of studies over the years have suggested that antihistamine-containing compounds do increase the viscosity of middle ear fluid and reduce the chances that such fluid will resolve either spontaneously or with medical treatment. At this time, I recommend using oral decongestants in lieu of antihistamine-decongestant compounds in children with middle ear effusions.

What about the usual oral antihistamine-decongestants?
The well-known over-the-counter "cold" medication compounds, Dimetapp and Triaminic, changed over the past years. The "Combat Methamphetamine Epidemic Act of 2005" reclassified pseudoephedrine, the decongestant used in both these products, as a Schedule Listed Chemical requiring behind-the-counter storage or locked cabinet storage in pharmacies, and the law required a limit on the amount any given consumer could purchase. As a result, the manufacturers of "cold" medications, fearing that parents wouldn't take the trouble to see the pharmacist for a effective form of their medications, reformulated Dimetapp and Triaminic and removed the "Sudafed" drug. They substituted "PE" or phenylephrine, a drug with similar medicinal properties to Sudafed but a worrisome characteristic: dosages of it which will clear the nose may produce cardiac toxicity. For this reason, the FDA banned the reformulated antihistamine decongestant products such as *Dimetapp Cold and Allergy* liquid, *Triaminic Cold and Allergy*

liquid, and *Benadryl D Allergy and Sinus* liquid for infants and removed these drugs from the recommended list for children 2 through 6 years of age.

The most effective readily available children's decongestant is *Children's Sudafed Decongestant Liquid*. This medication must be administered 3 to 4 times per day. Dosing for children 24 pounds and above is 1 teaspoon for each 24 pounds. The dosing is reduced for children under 24 pounds, and a chart of dosages for children from 14 to 48 pounds may be found in the **Appendix**.

Topical decongestants:
If your infant or toddler is already receiving maximal doses of oral decongestants or oral antihistamine-decongestant yet the nose is draining and remains partially or completely blocked due to congestion, you will need to escalate the program to include a topical decongestant. Also, if your child's nose seems decongested but you suspect that post-nasal drainage is driving nighttime coughing, you will need a topical decongestant.

For infants, I recommend the use of *Little Noses Decongestant Nose Drops*, which contains 1/8% *phenylephrine*, a topical version of the same decongestant that I have just panned for oral use. It is extremely effective and safe when used topically. For children two years or older, I suggest the use of *Neo-Synephrine Mild Strength* nasal spray containing phenylephrine 1/4%. Children 6 years and older may use the longer acting agent Afrin. As with the oral decongestant, begin with a single dose of the spray at bedtime. If needed, add up to three more doses of *Little Noses Decongestant Drops* or *Mild Neo-Synephrine Nasal Spray*. For older children, use *Afrin* twice to three times daily.

The topical decongestants cause the small blood vessels feeding the nasal linings to constrict, and this action leads to very rapid shrinkage of the intranasal linings. Unfortunately, this type of medication, if used repeatedly for many weeks, will itself irritate the nasal linings leading to the *rebound effect*. This phenomenon has mistakenly been labeled a nose drop "addiction."

Use of the sprays over a 4 to 7 day period during the active phase of a "cold" is safe and well tolerated. As many as eight recent studies demonstrate that topical nasal decongestant sprays such as *Afrin* may be used for as 3 weeks before producing significant nasal lining irritation. Before instilling any medicated nasal spray, use a spray of saline to cleanse the nasal linings in order to improve absorption of the medication. This is similar to power washing your house before painting it.

Topical steroids:
The nasal lining swelling caused by viral infections, bacterial infections, allergies, and even by irritating inhaled agents may take an extended period of time to resolve. One antidote to this problem is treatment with a topical nasal steroid, an optional, prescription-only ingredient in the **SADDS** recipe. I realize that the word **steroid** immediately raises concerns in the minds of parents because we all know that steroids are powerful medications. Despite these concerns, let me reassure you that the latest generation of topical steroids has an impressive safety record due to very low absorption into the body proper. These medications include *Nasonex*, *Flonase*, and *Veramyst*. They are usually sprayed into each nasal cavity once or twice a day following a spray of saline. Reaching a maximal effect when significant tissue swelling is present may require weeks to months of administration.

Although these medications are safe, I continue to recommend minimizing their use, particularly in my youngest patients. As is the case for all medications, timing is everything, and timely use of topical nasal steroids can reduce the need for their continuation. With that in mind, let's talk about timing their use.

Topical nasal steroids effectively drive shrinkage and normalization of nasal linings that are swollen following the acute phase of "colds." I suggest beginning a 7 to 10 day course of a topical nasal steroid on day 7 of a "cold," at a time when the child's immune system has already mounted a response to the virus.

Don't use them at the beginning of the "cold" for two reasons. First of all, topical steroids are not capable decongestants, and they do not work well to acutely shrink the nasal linings during the first days of a "cold." Of more importance is the fact that topical steroids slow the body's immune elimination of the "cold" viruses. Studies have demonstrated that live viruses shed longer from nasal cavities being treated with topical nasal steroids at the beginning of "colds." Use of such agents may prolong "cold" symptoms and increase the chance of a secondary bacterial infection.

For acute decongestion, parents should use oral decongestants, oral antihistamine-decongestants, and topical decongestants, the mainstay medications of the **SADDS** decongestion recipe. Begin use of any topical nasal steroids only at day 7 or later after the onset of the "cold."

The table below reviews my decongestion recipe:

Table:
Decongestion Recipe for Recurrent Otitis Media:
The SADDS Recipe

Step	Rationale	Use	Ingredient/ Measure
Saline mist nasal irrigation	Moisturization of linings and mucus, cleansing away contaminants	2 sprays in each nostril 3 times a day; more often during "colds."	Simply Saline Aerosol; also aerosol versions of Ocean, Little Noses, and store brands.

Oral Anti-inflammatory Medications	Inhibition of tissue swelling and secretion production within the nasal cavities, middle ears, sinuses, and throat cavities.	3 doses/day	*Infants, Children, Adolescents*: Ibuprofen as *Advil, Motrin,* or store brands.
Oral Decongestant Medications	Acute shrinkage and some drying of nasal linings.	Short acting agents using 2 to 4 doses/day	*Infants*: Children's Sudafed Nasal Decongestion Liquid *Children*: Children's Sudafed Nasal Decongestion Liquid *Adolescents*: Sudafed short and long-acting formulations.
Topical Decongestants	Powerful short-term shrinkage and drying of nasal linings.	**Short acting agents:** 3 to 4 doses/day. **Long acting agent:** 2 to 3 times a day. *Note*: Always administer saline mist nasal irrigation prior to a medicated nasal spray.	*Infants :* Little Noses Decongestant Drops (1/8%) *Older Infants and Children* (2-6 yrs): Mild Neo-Synephrine Nasal Spray (1/4%) *Older Children and Adolescents*: Afrin Nasal Decongestant

Topical Steroids (optional, prescription ingredient)	Long-term shrinkage and drying of swollen and chronically infected or inflamed nasal linings. Effectively returns nasal linings inflamed by viral or bacterial infections, allergies, or airborne irritants to normal.	Effective as "punctuating" course following each "cold." Avoid initiation of therapy during the first 7 days of a "cold." *Note*: Always administer saline mist nasal irrigation prior to a medicated nasal spray.	*Infants and Younger Children* (0-4 yrs): *Nasonex, Veramyst* twice a day beginning day 7 and use for 10 days. *Children and Adolescents* (4 yrs and above: *Flonase* twice a day beginning day 7 and use for 10 days.

INFECTION PREVENTION

The second portion of the VIP recipe for treatment of recurring ear infections is targeted toward infection prevention. In the first phase of the program, our goal is to stop the apparent "yo-yo" pattern of Mikey's infections. That is, we want to assure that Mikey will not quickly redevelop a middle ear infection once he finishes his current course of a "heavy hitter" antibiotic.

Relapsing infections occur in part because the linings of a child's middle ear spaces, nasal cavities, and adenoidal craters are often coated with a thin film of mucus, a so-called **biofilm**, which encases bacteria and holds these "bugs" in a form of suspended animation. We are currently only in the early stages of understanding what causes the formation and eradication of biofilms, but our knowledge is growing. My clinical observations suggest that viral upper respiratory infections seem to trigger the reactivation of these "sleeping" bacteria, allowing them to reactivate and proliferate.

My experience has shown that a combination of consistent, gradually diminishing antibiotic coverage, avoidance of new infections using episodic antibiotic prophylaxis, and aggressive management of ill-timed upper respiratory infections works best for stopping a run of persistent or rapidly relapsing infections.

**Eradicate residual infection
with continuous antibiotic prophylaxis:**
The first step in stabilizing Mikey's middle ear status is the continuing use of an antibiotic for at 20 to 30 days, the use of so-called continuous antibiotic prophylaxis. This type of program, using once-a-day low dose antibiotic, is often used by pediatricians for several months and sometimes for an entire winter. Long term, low dose antibiotic usage has been implicated in the development of resistant bacteria within the community.

I have developed a different approach to using continuous antibiotic prophylaxis which avoids this resistance-induction issues. My regimen for each child is highly variable depending on his or her previous "rap sheet" of ear infections and the child's social history including numbers of young siblings and attendance at day care or pre-school. For the toughest cases, I will recommend that the child take a full therapeutic dose of one of the stronger antibiotics for up to 4 weeks. Usually, though, I will prescribe an antibiotic of moderate strength at a full therapeutic level for 7 to 10 days and then drop the level down to half-strength for the next two to three weeks. Should the child develop nasal congestion and drainage either due to a "cold" or teething, I suggest that the antibiotic be increased back to full strength for a one week period.

In Mikey's case, I will follow the Augmentin with a higher dose of a moderate antibiotic such as trimethoprim-sulfa (Bactrim or Septra) for 7 to 10 days at full strength, that is twice daily, and then recommend once a day therapy for the another 3 to 4 weeks before his next visit with me. During this antibiotic treatment phase, it is mandatory that Mikey's nasal cavities be kept clean and clear using any or all ingredients of my decongestion program. As the course of antibiotics helps Mikey's immune system vanquish infection and bacterial overgrowth in all sites, the requirement for decongestion will diminish and so too should the use of decongesting medications except saline mist nasal irrigation. Should Mikey be unfortunate enough to develop an upper respiratory infection such as a nasty "cold" during this treatment period, his parents will increase the antibiotic dose back up to a twice daily therapeutic level while ramping up his decongestion program. Stay tuned for more about this special recipe to be used during "colds." You will see it in use again and again.

Avoid sources of new infection:
When fighting persisting or relapsing infections, the last thing that a child's already stressed immune system needs is yet another infection. One key to infection prevention is avoiding those people and places where infections "live." Large day care centers are breeding grounds for infections. The population of kids is large enough that someone in contact with your child is either becoming sick or is sick, and therefore capable of infecting your child. Studies have shown that when 5 or more infants, toddlers, or younger children play together, the incidence of upper respiratory infection escalates. While the average child will develop 5 to 7 "colds" or upper respiratory infections between October and May of each year, children in day care and pre-school have more of these infections and their infections often last longer.

Ideally, acutely ill children should remain home and not attend their day care center or pre-school. Unfortunately, this may not be practical, but some centers do isolate children with upper respiratory infections and employ other maneuvers to prevent infection transmission.

Day care centers can reduce the incidence of upper respiratory infections in their attendees by employing hand washing, saline nasal sprays, and humidification. To reduce the chances of hand-to-hand followed by hand-to-mouth spread of contaminated mucus, all kids in the group should wash their hands *at least once for every two hours of play*. Another helpful maneuver, particular during the colder, drier autumn and winter weather when each child's nasal linings dry out and "crust out" quickly, is the repeated use of a saline nasal spray during each session. As a minimum, hand washing and use of the saline nasal spray should definitely occur immediately following each play session. When heat is on in the classroom, humidification to 40-50% relative humidity using a warm mist humidifier will maintain respiratory linings in a healthy state. I suggest to Mikey's parents that his day-care center and the room where the playgroup meets in each home be equipped with a humidifier, especially in homes with forced hot air heat. This will help Mikey and his peers maintain clean and naturally decongested middle ear linings.

Besides his participation in day care three times weekly, Mikey attends informal play groups on a regular basis. When Mikey has an active "cold" or other symptoms of a significant upper respiratory infection such as coughing, wheezing, apparent throat soreness, or hoarseness, he should not attend. The other children in his playgroup should follow the same rules, and Mikey's parents will be having a discussion with the other parents in his group. Similarly, if a sibling or parent of a child in the group is ill, the group should not meet at that "sick home."

Mikey is, so far, an only child. If your child has older siblings, they are only too happy to bring germs home for your infant or toddler to fully enjoy. If that occurs, try to isolate your sick children, avoid close contact between them and the healthy kids, and insist on good hand washing along with liberal use of saline mist irrigation by all members of the household. Oh, yes, be certain that each member of the family has his or her own bottle of saline.

Another source of infection is the pacifier, and population studies in Scandinavia reveal that children using pacifiers experience significantly more bouts of otitis media. Pacifiers get passed around and they transmit germs from child to child in the home and in day care centers. Furthermore, an infant's continual sucking on the pacifier serves to reduce middle ear pressure which, in turn, will draw possibly contaminated nasal and throat mucus into the middle ear space. I, as well as many pediatricians, recommend that parents stop their infant's continual use of pacifiers after 6 months of age and eliminate the use of pacifiers before and during sleep by 10 months of age.

Boost your child's immunity:
It is important to keep your child's preventive immunization program up-to-date. The most recent addition to the treatment for infants with recurring ear infections is a vaccine called *Prevnar*. This "shot" generates immunity against selected types of the *pneumococcus*, one family of bacteria implicated as a common cause for recurrent otitis media. This vaccine only protects against common subgroups of *pneumococci*, but they are the ones most likely to be resistant to our best antibiotics. The current literature suggests that the vaccine eliminates close to 60% of those otitis media episodes due to the classes of pneumococcus included in the vaccine. Since only about 40 to 50 percent of otitis media episodes are caused by pneumococci, *Prevnar* has driven an overall reduction in ear infections of 20 to 25 percent. These infections, though, are the most difficult to treat with currently available antibiotics. As a result, the number of children having ear surgery for recurrent or persistent ear infections has diminished.

Although we have been able to vaccinate older children against pneumococci for many years, the *Prevnar* vaccine now permits vaccination of infants. The *Prevnar* vaccine binds pneumococcal antigens to immunogenic proteins, and this novel presentation permits infants, who have weak immune systems, to mount an adequate reaction to the pneumococcal antigens and to produce protective antibodies. *Prevnar* vaccination requires 3 to 4 doses for maximal effectiveness, and you should be certain that your child completes the immunization program outlined by your pediatrician.

For older children and adolescents who never received *Prevnar*, the time-tested polysaccharide-bound pneumococcal vaccine called *Pneumovax* is available and should be administered according to the recommended schedules. This vaccine immunizes children and adolescents 2 years and older to multiple antigenic varieties of pneumococci.

Stay tuned for information regarding the necessity for re-immunization, as these vaccines, like most others, will likely not confer permanent immunity. Fortunately, nearly all children tend to outgrow ear infection problems when they reach late adolescence. Unfortunately, the same cannot be said for sinusitis problems. That is a topic for another day.

Infants with recurrent otitis media should also be considered for influenza vaccination. Upper respiratory infections driven by susceptible classes of influenza are preventable, and every little bit helps. Ask your child's pediatrician about obtaining these useful immunizations.

Another maneuver that enhances your child's natural immunity is breast-feeding. While antibodies passed from the mother via the placental circulation power the newborn's immune system, after about 6 months those antibodies are depleted. Breast-feeding provides a new supply of antibodies to supplement those under construction by the infant's own fledgling immune system. Studies suggest that regular breast-feeding may diminish a child's incidence of otitis media by 25%. Unfortunately, by the time most new moms read this paragraph, they have stopped breast-feeding prematurely or elected never to begin it. Please pass the word.

There are rumblings about that certain probiotics can also stimulate the immune system. The World Health Organization defines probiotics as "live microorganisms which, when administered in adequate amounts, confer a health benefit on the host." The best examples are live culture lactobacilli found in yogurt and in other preparations including *Culturelle*. The jury is still out, but initial studies hint that regular ingestion of such foods or over-the-counter sources of lactobacilli will help increase host resistance to infection.

Prevent viral "colds" from igniting bacterial ear infections: Given Murphy's Law, many infants and children will develop "colds" or nasal congestion due to teething or allergies during the period of continuous antibiotic prophylaxis. As noted above, during these episodes I ask parents to increase the antibiotic dose back up to full-strength.

Currently, Mikey is using the short-term, low dose continuous antibiotic prophylaxis with the time-honored antibiotic called *Bactrim*. It also goes by its generic name trimethoprim-sulfa or by another brand name *Septra*. Should he develop a "cold," teething associated nasal congestion, or severe allergy-driven nasal congestion, I have instructed his folks to increase his frequency of *Bactrim* administration from once to twice a day, a full therapeutic dose.

Table:
Infection Prevention Recipe for Recurrent Otitis Media

Step	Rationale	Use	Ingredient/Measure
Eradicate Residual Infection and Stop "Yo-yo" Infections using Continuous Antibiotic Prophylaxis	Use of **continuous antibiotic prophylaxis to** eliminate bacterial organisms colonizing the middle ear spaces, nasal linings, and throat linings including the adenoids.	**Continuous antibiotic,** extended course. Begin at normal therapeutic dose; proceed to lower the dose to half-strength. Dose increase during "colds," teething, allergic nasal congestion. Use antibiotic with maximal nasal decongestion [SADDS recipe] using saline nasal irrigation, anti-inflammatory agents, oral and topical decongestants, possible topical nasal steroids.	• Use mild and moderate class antibiotics such as amoxicillin and Bactrim (trimethoprim-sulfa); use stronger antibiotics as needed. • For cleansing, use saline nasal spray 3 times a day or more. For decongestion, use oral decongestants such as Sudafed, topical decongestants such as Little Noses Decongestant Drops, Mild Neo-Synephrine Nasal Spray, or Afrin. For more rapid normalization of nasal linings following "colds," topical nasal steroids such as Nasonex, Flonase, or Veramyst.
Avoid Infection Sources: Day Care	Prefer day care settings with fewer children (5 or fewer), well children, and infection transmission avoidance policies.	• Sitters in child's home • Home day care with 5 or fewer children better than center day care. • Infection prevention maneuvers.	• Sitters or home day care. • Exclude sick children. • Use saline mist nasal irrigation and humidification. • Use frequent hand washing.

Avoid Infection Sources: Play Groups	Prefer playgroup settings with fewer children, well children, and infection transmission avoidance policies.	• Play groups with 5 or fewer children. • Infection prevention maneuvers.	• Exclude sick children. • Use saline mist nasal irrigation and humidification. • Use frequent hand washing.
Avoid Infection Sources: Siblings	Prevent siblings from transmitting upper respiratory infections.	• Isolate sibs who are ill. • Infection prevention maneuvers.	• Avoidance of hand-to-hand contact. • Frequent hand washing. • Use of saline mist nasal irrigation and humidification.
Avoid Infection Sources: Pacifiers	Eliminating pacifier use reduces ear infections 33-50%.	• Pacifiers pass "germs" from child to child. • Pacifiers encourage sucking, swallowing, and produce negative middle ear pressures.	If at all, only permit infants over 6 months to use while falling asleep, discontinue all use for infants at 10 months of age

Boost Your Child's Immunity	• Immunizations to prevent ear infections cause by specific bacteria and to prevent severe viral upper respiratory infections. • Breast feeding reduces ear infections by 25%	• Anti-pneumococcal vaccine. • Influenza vaccine. • Breast feeding	• *Prevnar* protein-conjugated anti-pneumococci vaccine for infants. • *Pneumovax* polysaccharide-bound anti-pneumococci vaccine for older children and selected adolescents. • Influenza vaccine. • Breast-feed as long as possible.
Prevent Viral "Colds" from Igniting Bacterial Ear Infections	Use of therapeutic level **episodic antibiotic prophylaxis** to prevent growth of bacterial middle ear organisms entering the middle ear spaces from the nasal cavities during vulnerable periods	Use of antibiotic daily at normal therapeutic doses **only** at times of nasal congestion including "colds", vigorous teething, significant allergic nasal congestion. Use antibiotic with and maximal nasal decongestion [SADD recipe] decongestants.	Milder or moderate antibiotics such as amoxicillin, Bactrim, and Cefzil; stronger antibiotics as needed. Frequent saline nasal spray; oral inflammatories such as Motrin or Advil, oral decongestants such as Sudafed, topical decongestants such as Mild Neo-Synephrine Nasal Spray or Afrin, optional use of "punctuating" courses of topical nasal steroids following each "cold"

Mikey returns

When I see an infant such as Mikey back in the office for a first follow up after beginning my regimens, the eardrums and, by proxy, the middle ear linings look considerably healthier. They are thinner and show fewer signs of inflammation. The child's nasal linings appear clean and less swollen.

At this point, in the interest of minimizing antibiotic use and giving Mikey's gastrointestinal system a break, it is time to transition him from continuous antibiotic prophylaxis to a program of episodic antibiotic prophylaxis. He will continue all regimens for ventilation and general infection prevention, but his parents will now only use a prophylactic antibiotic when and if he develops certain conditions that predispose to the development of the next ear infection. These include the common cold, teething with nasal symptoms, or escalating nasal congestion due to allergies or other airborne irritants. When these events occur, Mikey will use my episodic antibiotic prophylaxis recipe, the **SAADD** recipe.

The Episodic Antibiotic Prophylaxis Recipe (SAADD Recipe) for Preventing Ear infections during "Colds"

My recipe for successful prevention of subsequent ear infections combines the proactive use of episodic antibiotic prophylaxis with maximal nasal decongestion. I call it the **SAADD recipe**.

Decode this acronym as follows:

S:	saline mist irrigation
A:	episodic antibiotic prophylaxis
A:	oral anti-inflammatory
D:	oral decongestant
D:	topical decongestant

Mikey will use this recipe whenever he develops an upper respiratory infection such as a "cold," significant nasal congestion in association with teething, or escalating nasal congestion and drainage in association with allergies.

Let's talk first about "colds." Mikey's parents tell me that they have rarely used medications to control his "cold" symptoms. They, as many other parents, take a conservative approach to treating this common malady: the less medication the better. Furthermore, they infrequently receive much guidance about how to treat "colds" from their childrens' pediatricians.

I too am in favor of minimizing the use of medications, but some *are* necessary. Strategy and timing are critical in order to get the *maximal* effect from the *minimal* amounts of medication and to keep your child breathing comfortably while preventing the common complications of "colds," ear infections, and sinus infections. The background and rationale for treating "colds" is outlined in the chapter entitled ***Recipes for Treating "Colds."*** You may choose to read this now or later.

If you chose to read the "cold" chapter, welcome back and excuse a small amount of repetition. As we move on, remember that the most critical part of "cooking" is learning to use the various medications and other ingredients in an organized and timely fashion in order to manage your child's "cold" like a virtuoso. The parents I have coached and who have successfully mastered use of my recipes would pass on the following recommendation: don't take a "wait and see" attitude when you spot the beginning of an upper respiratory infection.

At the first sign of "cold" symptoms, *immediately* begin the antibiotic and the decongestion program. If you start earlier, you *will* be able to stop earlier. If you wait too long, mucus will accumulate and clog the nasal passages including the critical vent ports for the ears and sinuses leading to bacterial infection and a prolonged course of antibiotics and decongestants. Be creative and experiment! *You* know your child best, and *you* can call the shots better than the professionals sitting miles away in their offices.

The centerpiece of the **SAADD** recipe for ear infection prevention is the strategic use of prophylactic antibiotics. Why, you might ask, do I recommend treating a viral infection with antibiotics? Conventional antibiotics do not kill viruses!

The last statement is true but not directly relevant. It turns out that most children's immune systems are fully capable of slowing and stopping the viral infection, often caused by adenoviruses and rhinoviruses. For this reason, most well-behaved and well-managed "colds" are over by 7 days following their start and not likely to lead to a middle ear infection or to a rhinosinusitis. On the other hand, if the cold" is not well-behaved or well-managed, if sneezing, coughing, and nose blowing abound, then viruses and bacteria are widely distributed and the nasal passages, the sinus cavities, and the middle ear spaces all become so boggy and swamp-like that a new set problems begins to emerge.

This new set of problems is bacterial in nature. Even though the viruses are dropping like flies at the hands of your child's white cell army, reinforcements for the viruses are emerging in the form of proliferating bacteria of three principal types: *streptococcus pneumoniae, hemophilus influenza*, and *moraxella catarrhalis*. We in the trade call these nasty bugs by nicknames: *pneumo* (pronounced nu-mo), *h-flu*, and *m-cat*. Unlike viruses, these bacteria often grow faster than your child's immune system can kill them. They grow in all of the boggy crevices within the middle ear spaces, within the nasal passages and sinuses, and within the throat including the adenoids and tonsils. They produce a potpourri of infections including ear infections, sinus infections, adenoid infections, tonsillitis, and bronchitis.

The reasons that some "colds" are total outlaws and others are well behaved include the development and strength of your child's immune system, your child's natural powers of decongestion, your child's pain threshold, and, of primary importance, how *you* manage the illness.

Once you begin the antibiotics, they should continue until the child's nasal congestion is gone. They need not be continued for a set 10-day period. Remember, in contrast to using antibiotics for treatment of, say, a strep throat, you are using them to prevent, not treat infection. They may be stopped when the danger has passed. Similarly, you will dial back the decongestion program when your child's congestion clears.

The best way to understand the **SAADD** recipe is to look at its day-by-day application during a typical "cold." The road map may be found in Table D. At the first sign of a "cold," begin the episodic antibiotic prophylaxis immediately. Since we use the mildest members of the antibiotic family, they must be started at the very onset of "cold" symptoms or when teething begins in order to have a strategic advantage. To do this, parents must have a supply of antibiotics as well as decongestants ready to go.

Since "colds" never begin at convenient times, I gave Mikey's folks a refillable prescription for a mild antibiotic such as amoxicillin or trimethoprim-sulfa, an antibiotic combo formerly marketed under the brand names *Bactrim* or *Septra*. I asked them to fill the prescription and to have the antibiotic ready for a "call to action."

Whenever I prescribe an antibiotic such as amoxicillin, which must be refrigerated and which has a limited life after reconstitution as a liquid, I ask the pharmacist to dispense the medication in the unmixed, powdered form. This may be stored at a controlled room temperature range for many months or even years. I also ask that the pharmacist provide pre-measured distilled water for use by mom and dad in preparing the suspension for use.

I instruct mom and dad to reconstitute the antibiotic powder by slowly pouring the provided distilled water into the bottle with the powder. I remind them to stop pouring after about one-quarter of the water has been added and swirl the bottle to mix the power with the available fluid. Continuing adding each additional 25% and repeat the mixing process until all of the liquid has been added and mixed in. Once the powder is reconstituted, the antibiotic may require refrigeration and its shelf life will likely be limited. The remainder of the antibiotic should be discarded after the "cold" is over, and a new supply of powdered antibiotic obtained to have on hand for the next upper respiratory infection.

Once the "cold" is off and running, all other medications should also begin. Use sufficient amounts of saline to keep your child's nasal passages clear and clean. Begin the anti-inflammatory ibuprofen, *Motrin*, *Advil* or the generic equivalent, and use doses of it 3 times a day for the entire 7 days of the "cold." Congestion and nasal drainage usually peak between days 3 to 5, and, during those days, your child will like require systemic and topical decongestants such as oral *Sudafed* and/or topical *Little Noses Decongestant Drops* for infants, *Mild Neo-Synephrine Nasal Spray* for children 2 years until 6 years of age, or *Afrin* for children 6 years and older in order to supplement the decongestant effects of the ibuprofen. Usually, by day 7 of the "cold," it is possible to stop the antibiotic coverage, the anti-inflammatory ibuprofen, and all decongestants.

Antibiotic overuse has already produced consequences. We are now fighting bacteria ever more resistant to stronger and stronger antibiotics. The use of episodic antibiotic prophylaxis, a short pulse of an effective antibiotic before the fact, prevents the need for a prolonged course of a stronger antibiotic to treat an established infection.

There are a number of fine points about treating "colds." Are discolored secretions a sign that the therapy is failing? When coughing occurs during a "cold," what does it mean and what should you do about it? Should you teach your child to blow his or her nose? Let me just get the answer to this last question off my chest now for the first time and repeat it as often as I can. ABSOLUTELY DO NOT BLOW THE NOSE! Nose blowing irritates nasal linings and may force infected mucus up into eustachian tubes and the sinus ventilation channels. If you treat the "cold" aggressively with the medications I have already discussed, nose blowing will be unnecessary. For more details about this and other tricks to fighting "colds," see the chapter *Recipes for Treating "Colds."*

Table:

Roadmap of the SAADD recipe:

Episodic Antibiotic Prophylaxis during "colds"

Day	Events	Treatment	Medication
1	• Sudden development of mild congestion • Clear nasal drainage	• First line antibiotic therapy as prophylaxis • Saline mist nasal irrigation Anti-inflammatory medication round the clock Oral and/or topical decongestants for marked initial congestion	• Amoxicillin, Bactrim, Cefzil • Simply Saline aerosol, Ocean saline aerosol, Little Noses saline aerosol • Motrin, Advil or generic ibuprofen • Sudafed by mouth, Little Noses Decongestant Drops*, Mild Neo-Synephrine Nasal Spray+, Afrin#
2	• Moderate congestion • More and thicker drainage	• Continue episodic antibiotic prophylaxis therapy • More frequent nasal saline • Continue anti-inflammatory medications • Oral/topical decongestant medications	• Continue antibiotic • More Simply Saline • Motrin, Advil or generic ibuprofen • Sudafed by mouth, Little Noses Decongestant Drops*, Mild Neo-Synephrine Nasal Spray+, Afrin#
3-5	• Intense congestion • Maximal drainage	• Continue episodic antibiotic prophylaxis therapy • Maximize nasal saline • Continue anti-inflammatory medications • Oral/topical decongestant medications	• Continue antibiotic • Maximal Simply Saline • Motrin, Advil or generic ibuprofen • Sudafed by mouth, Little Noses Decongestant Drops*, Mild Neo-Synephrine Nasal Spray+, Afrin#

RECURRENT OTITIS

7	• Waning congestion • Waning drainage	• Stop first-line antibiotic • Less nasal saline • Return to day 2 or day 1 decongestant implementation	• Stop antibiotic • Reduce saline • Motrin, Advil or the generic ibuprofen
≥7	• Minimal congestion • No drainage	• Saline back to baseline administration	

* - for infants; + - for younger children; # - for children 6 yrs. and over

Some children experience a very slow reduction of their nasal lining swelling following each "cold." For those kids, I recommend an alternate conclusion to each use of the **SAADDS** recipe: a short course of topical nasal steroids. This should be started on day 7 of the "cold" in order that the steroids, locally immunosuppressive, will not interfere with the body's natural immune elimination of the virus. The topical nasal steroids are continued for 7 to 10 days and then discontinued. This alternate scenario is shown in the following table.

Table:

Roadmap of a SAADDS alternative strategy for managing persisting nasal congestion

Day	Events	Treatment	Medication
7	• Persisting congestion • Clear drainage	• Begin topical nasal steroid once* or twice+# a day • Stop first-line antibiotic • Nasal saline 2 to 3 times a day	• Begin Nasonex*+ or Flonase+# once or twice a day • Stop episodic antibiotic prophylaxis • Simply Saline 2 to 3 times a day • Sudafed and/or Little Noses Decongestant Drops, Mild Neo-Synephrine Nasal Spray, or Afrin
≥7	• Minimal congestion • No drainage	• Continue topical nasal steroid for 6 to 9 more days • Continue twice daily saline mist administration for duration of topical nasal steroid administration • Stop decongestants	• Continue Nasonex*+ or Flonase+# once or twice a day for 6 to 9 more days • Simply Saline or another saline aerosol 2 times a day

* - for infants; + - for younger children; # - for children 6 yrs and over

We have been assuming so far that, with maximal nasal decongestion, we can tame Mikey's "colds," and, with the timely use of antibiotic prophylaxis, we can prevent them from spawning secondary infections in the ear, nose, and sinuses. Sometimes, the "weaker" antibiotics that we use for prophylaxis are insufficient to prevent bacterial overgrowth as the viral phase of the "cold" is resolving. This may be particularly true in day care attendees such as Mikey, since he may contract particularly resistant forms of *pneumo*, *h-flu*, and *m-cat* from his peers.

The signs of this problem are the appearance and persistence after one week of discolored nasal secretions with continuing nasal congestion and post-nasal drainage. This indicates bacterial overgrowth in the nasal cavities and sinuses. When this occurs, I suggest that a child's parents confer with me.

If there is no clinical history which mandates an in-person examination, I will customarily order a stronger antibiotic to "rescue" the patient. On the other hand, if a child has a history of this situation occurring repeatedly or if a child develops more worrisome signs such as fever, ear pain, headache, throat soreness, and cough, I will invite a visit for an exam and a possible nasopharyngeal culture.

Table : Roadmap of a SAADD alternative strategy for eradicating a developing bacterial nasal/sinus infection

Day	Events	Treatment	Medication
5-6	• Persisting nasal congestion • Discolored drainage after day 7 following onset of "cold" as sign of impending bacterial intranasal and sinus infection	• Begin stronger antibiotic as "rescue" medication • Stop milder prophylactic antibiotic • Continue max nasal saline for duration of "rescue" antibiotic • Use day 3-4 decongestant routine with systemic and topical decongestants for duration of "rescue" antibiotic	•Begin Omnicef or Augmentin • Simply Saline • Little Noses Decongestant Drops*, Mild Neo-Synephrine Nasal Spray+; or Afrin nasal spray# • Sudafed Children's Nasal Decongestant

* - for infants; + - for younger children; # - for children 6 yrs and over

Mikey almost "crashes"

Mikey's dad calls one day in early winter to tell me that he believes the **SAADD** program is failing. After four successive "colds" that responded beautifully to the regimen with initially Cefzil and subsequently amoxicillin as the episodic antibiotic prophylaxis agent, Mikey is not doing well. His two most recent "colds" failed to resolve on the first line antibiotic and required "rescue" courses of second line antibiotics.

To be certain that this phenomenon does not repeat, I escalate his episodic antibiotic prophylaxis agent up to the next antibiotic group. He returns to the moderate antibiotic Cefzil successfully for two subsequent "cold" cycles, and I then recommend that he return to the use of amoxicillin for the remainder of the colder weather.

About ambush or "guerilla otitis" media

Most bouts of otitis media in infants and children occur during "colds," that is viral infections of the nasal cavities and upper throat. Other children also develop otitis media following the nasal symptoms in association with teething. Mikey developed a few bouts of otitis media without "colds" or teething, and some children always develop otitis media without any of these symptoms or associations. This situation makes it difficult if not impossible for parents to know when to start a child's episodic antibiotic prophylaxis.

Actually, there is almost always SOME identifiable driver for ear infections. On careful parent questioning, most infants without obvious "colds" preceding their ear infections do have other upper respiratory problems rather than the stereotypical nasal symptoms. For instance, a child may have isolated coughing or a sore throat.

For such children, in order for episodic antibiotic prophylaxis agent to get the necessary advantage and prevent acute otitis media episodes, we broaden the indications for starting them. I ask parents to begin the antibiotic at the first sign of coughing or fever in addition to the first signs of "colds" or teething. With some infants, I suggest antibiotic initiation for ear pulling or the onset of behavior that characteristically heralds their ear infections. In the situations where nasal symptoms are absent, parents need not begin the maximal nasal decongestion regimen yet should continue the prophylactic antibiotics for the duration of the triggering symptoms and for at least one week.

Those children who develop acute middle ear infections without any upper respiratory infection trigger, may be harboring middle ear fluid which is difficult for their pediatricians to see with an otoscope. This fluid contained the bacteria which, at any time, may suddenly begin to grow.

Mikey "graduates"

As I see Mikey back periodically through the late winter and early spring, he weathers many "colds" without the development of any otitis media episodes. His second birthday passes. With the coming of warmer weather, I suggest to his folks that we back off the use of antibiotics. We modify his **VIP Program** for "colds" by eliminating the first "sniffle" use of antibiotic prophylaxis. With each cold, he continues to ramp up his use of saline and begin maximal nasal decongestion, but he uses no antibiotics. If his "cold" symptoms linger into the second week making it more likely that the "cold" will seed his ears or sinuses, we will begin the use of the prophylactic antibiotic. Initially, I give his parents an open prescription for an antibiotic but later ask them to call if his "colds" fail to remain "well-behaved." Since all continues to go well and since he is developing excellent expressive language, I discharge him from my surveillance program. If his speech were suboptimal, I would refer him for a complete audiometric evaluation.

CHECKLIST: *The VIP Program for Recurrent Otitis Media*
VENTILATION:
  Cleansing:
      Saline mist irrigation
      Humidification
      Air cleansing
      Prevent stomach reflux
      Consider and treat allergies
  Decongestion:
      Saline mist irrigation
      Oral decongestants
      Oral anti-inflammatories
      Topical decongestants
      Topical nasal steroids

INFECTION PREVENTION:
  Clear residual bacterial infection:
      Therapeutic antibiotic treatment
      Continuous antibiotic prophylaxis
  Avoid infection sources:
      Healthy playmates
      Healthy older siblings
      Small day care peer group
      Hand washing
      Humidification
      Pacifier elimination
  Keep immunizations up to date:
      Anti-pneumococcal vaccine (Prevnar)
      Anti-hemophilus influenzae vaccine (HiB)
      Influenza vaccine
  Treat upper respiratory infections:
      SADDS maximal nasal decongestion program with
          possible use of topical nasal steroids
  Prevent bacterial superinfections:
      Continuous antibiotic prophylaxis
      Episodic antibiotic prophylaxis - SAADD

4 -- Recipes for Persisting Otitis Media

Meet Michele
Michele's First Visit
The SuperVIP Program for Persistent Otitis Media
    SuperVentilation or Steroid Ventilation
    Infection Processing
Michele returns
Michele "graduates"
VIP Program for Persisting Otitis Media at a Glance

Most infants and children with recurrent ear infections tend to initially clear acute infections after treatment, but, in some children with successive infections, it becomes more and more difficult to do so. Repeated ear infections lead to swelling of the middle ear and eustachian tube linings. As a result, air cannot reenter the ear, and the middle ear space frequently retains infection and fluid. Persistent and rapidly relapsing ear infections become more common.

The effective elimination of such persistent infection with medical therapy alone is more challenging. It requires the application of my **VIP Program** and its component recipes utilizing some special tweaks and twists. To better understand my approach to this problem, let's meet Michele, a toddler with ear infections that just won't quit.

Meet Michele

Michele is an adorable toddler who bounced into my office for her first visit at 20 months of age. Her "rap sheet" of ear infections revealed a list of 10 over the preceding year with a pattern of severity escalation. They began when she entered day care.

Initially, her infections cleared on a single course of antibiotic, but, as time wore on, two courses of antibiotics were necessary and the interval between infections began to dwindle. For the six weeks preceding her visit with me, her latest infections had failed to respond completely to any antibiotic. She had been treated with medications of increasing strength, with the most recent use of heavy hitters including *Ceftin* and *Augmentin Extra Strength*. Her parents were at their wits' end, since Michele's sleeping patterns had deteriorated to the point that she was awake and they were up with her most of the night, every night. Her pediatrician called me with the request that I see her the next day and consider ventilating her ears with the placement of tympanostomy tubes as soon as that could be arranged.

Michele's First Visit

I brought Michele in the next day for a visit. Her parents, Jon and Alyse, were very friendly but clearly very fatigued and frankly scared by the prospect that their baby might be visiting the operating room within the week. Michele herself seemed in no distress: she was not running a fever and did not appear ill. Despite her many ear infections, she was quite responsive to sounds. She seemed to be almost hypersensitive to loud noise and music, not an unusual situation in children with middle ear problems, as their swollen middle ear linings tend to distort sound and make even melodious sounds very noticeable but annoying.

She was on day 9 of the *Augmentin ES*, and her ear examination revealed very thickened and chronically inflamed tympanic membranes. There was milky fluid in her middle ear spaces. They were not bulging. Tympanograms failed to reveal any middle ear air. Her nasal linings were swollen, and she did have evidence of infection within her nasal cavities. Her throat examination was normal except for evidence of purulent post-nasal drainage.

Michele's history and physical exam are typical of infants with persistent otitis media. Her rapidly recurring and now persisting otitis media signals two ear problems and possible nasal issues: excessive thickening of her middle ear and eustachian tube linings and the presence of "industrial strength" bacterial organisms likely resistant to conventional antibiotics; chronic nasal and nasopharyngeal lining edema and/or infection.

Michele's predicament is typical of most infants and toddlers with persisting otitis media. She has been exposed to nasty bacteria in the day care setting that were only partially eradicated by the mild antibiotics she received. The linings of her middle ear and mastoid spaces became swollen and the spaces themselves polluted. Her nasal problems, the presence of swollen linings and mucus sludge, compounded her ventilation and infection problems by preventing air from readily entering her eustachian tubes and also by acting as a source of infection. Persistent otitis media problems are living testimony to the biologic truism that lining swelling leads to infection AND infection leads to lining swelling.

The Super VIP Recipe for Persistent Otitis Media

From reading the previous chapter about recurrent otitis media, you will recall that my **VIP** program for managing ear infections is an acronym which stands for **ventilation and infection prevention**. When dealing with persisting otitis media, the program must be modified to deal with the additional challenges. I call this program my **SVIP**, my **Super VIP program** or my VIP program on steroids, literally and figuratively.

The SVIP master recipe is, as before, two individual but interrelated recipes, one for **Super or Steroid-assisted Ventilation (SV)** and the other for **Infection Processing (IP)** as well as infection prevention. This program has a number of "industrial strength" features, necessary due to the presence of pre-existing infection and its ravages.

SuperVENTILATION

My **SuperVentilation** program has several unique components in addition to the elements we have already discussed under the headings of cleansing and decongestion. The cleansing recipe is similar to that for recurrent ear infections with greater intensity, while the decongestion recipe is turbo-charged with steroids, both taken internally and applied topically on accessible nasal linings.

CLEANSING
Let's take a look at the components do the **SVIP** cleansing recipe:

Saline mist irrigation:
I can't say it often enough: instillation of over-the-counter saline spray is the single best cleanser for the nose. The saline mist is available in an aerosol sprayers as *Simply Saline, Ocean, and Little Noses.* I counsel against the use of saline in squeeze bottles as releasing he compressed container following application of the saline vacuums contaminated material off the tip of the nozzle into the bottle. Pump type dispensers are safer but not as contamination-proof as the aerosol canisters.

Children with significant nasal lining swelling should receive the saline spray using one or two sprays in each nostril three to six times a day. Let the mist cover the linings and do not suction the saline back out the front of the nose or encourage your child to blow the nose. These maneuvers will drive contaminated material from the back of the nose and from the adenoidal region into the "cleaner" front portions of the nose. Nasal secretions were meant to go backward: the floor of the nose is banked to the back rather than to the front of the nose, and none of us are born with gutters and downspouts beneath our nostrils.

Humidification:
Normal relative humidity, in the 40 to 45 percent range, is especially critical for children such as Michele, who are fighting excessive nasal lining swelling. Use a humidity gauge, a hygrometer, to check the humidity level and to help you set the humidity control on your humidifier. An inexpensive mechanical model is available at most Ace or TruValue hardware stores for about $8 to $10 US. More accurate but also more expensive electronic versions usually sell for about $10-30 US.

Cold or warm? I recommend the use of a **warm mist humidifier**, safer as it delivers water into the air as vaporized water molecules and not as droplets. Cold mist units aerosolize the reservoir water into droplets of moderate size. Bacteria or molds cannot piggyback on water molecules, but they can travel in water droplets. Infants such as Michele, who are already fighting infection, cannot tolerate contamination by the air they are breathing. To better circulate moisturized air from any humidifier around your child's room, use a safety fan with soft rubber blades to blow across the outflow nozzle of your humidifier. The fan is also a safety feature since it cools the vapor coming from the humidifier by mixing it with room air.

Are ultrasonic humidifiers safe where cold mist ones are not? The simple answer is a resounding NO! The ultrasonic unit "weaponizes" rather than merely aerosolizing the water, and the resulting droplets are small enough to travel into your child's lungs and trigger pneumonia.

Air cleansing:
No smoking of any kind, and avoid using "smoky" units of any kind including wood-burning stoves or fireplaces. Clean the house while your child is away from the action. Given the persistence of the child's ear and nasal problems, strict adherence to these guidelines is essential.

Stop stomach reflux:
Many children with persisting ear infections and nasal lining swelling experience both in association with black flow of stomach contents into their throats. This so-called **extra-esophageal reflux** produces nasal congestion and drainage, swelling of the adenoids, and eustachian tube malfunction. The physical signs of such reflux include chronic redness and "bumpy" lining swellings of the throat and voice box.

Controlling extra-esophageal reflux disease always requires special feeding strategies and may require acid suppression therapy. Avoid feeding your infant or child just before bedtime or a nap. Allow 60 to 90 minutes between feedings and sleeping in order to permit the stomach to completely empty before your child lies down. Try to compartmentalize feeding to other parts of the day.

If you wish to give your child a security "nightcap" or a middle of the night drink, give water in the bottle or sippy cup. The water, in contrast to milk or formula, will not induce stomach acid production. If you must feed just before bed or nap, maintain an upright position as sleep comes on by placing your child in a swing or car seat. After 60 to 90 minutes, transfer the child to the crib or bed.

If the child experiences persisting symptoms suggesting reflux or if the child's throat appears inflamed as the result of reflux, more aggressive diagnostic efforts are necessary. A direct examination of the lower throat and voice box using a fiberoptic endoscope may be useful in the search for the "footprints" of reflux in such children. Once reflux is confirmed, more aggressive medical therapy may be necessary. This includes acid suppression therapy using medications including histamine receptor antagonists such as *Zantac* and *Axid* or proton-pump inhibitors such as *Prevacid* and *Nexium*.

Identify and treat allergies:

The presence of persisting ear infections in the company of chronic or recurrent nasal congestion may indicate that a child has hypersensitivities to environmental agents. You, as a parent, are in a better position to make this diagnosis on clinical grounds than your child's pediatrician or even an allergist. The gradual onset of nasal congestion, sneezing, coughing, and itchy eyes after certain environmental exposures or at certain times of year may suggest the presence of allergies. Look for reactions while you are sweeping or dusting, while your child is playing around cats or dogs, or while your child is spending time out of doors near flowers, freshly cut grass, or weeds. The risk of allergy in your child is significantly higher if one or both parents currently have allergies or had a history of them as children.

If your child's clinical symptoms only suggest seasonal allergies, a formal allergy evaluation is not absolutely necessary. The time of year during which the symptoms appear will suggest the offending agents. Treatment may commence using rationales and recipes discussed in the chapter entitled *Recipes for Allergies*. If there is evidence of allergic nasal reactions for more than 4 months of the year, I recommend consideration of a formal allergy consultation with appropriate skin testing. This will pinpoint the culprits and suggest strategic and proactive therapeutic measures to neutralize them.

If an allergy evaluation yields negative results, your child may be suffering from non-allergic chronic rhinitis and rhinosinusitis. This is a complicated and poorly understood entity. The continuing nasal congestion, predominately posterior nasal drainage, secondary airway disorders such as asthma or asthma exacerbation, and eustachian tube dysfunction are caused by chronic inflammation of a child's nasal and sinus linings. This inflammation occurs as the results of physical assaults on your child's nasal and throat linings by viruses, bacteria, fungi, and even by contaminants in the air. I discuss this issue in more detail in *Recipes for Allergies*.

Table:
Cleansing Recipe for Persistent Otitis Media

Step	Rationale	Use	Ingredient/Measure
Saline mist nasal irrigation	Moisturization of linings and mucus, cleansing away contaminants.	2 sprays in each nostril 4 to 6 times a day.	Saline aerosol units such as Simply Saline, Ocean, Little Noses; pump versions of all products less ideal but preferred to squeeze bottles due to contamination
Humidification	Moisturization of linings and mucus to obtain humidity level of 40-45%.	While sleeping and napping but as often as possible.	Warm mist humidifier: Vicks, Honeywell, Holmes
Air cleansing	Air contaminated with irritants and allergens leads to nasal, throat, eustachian tube, and middle ear lining swelling.	All day, every day.	• NO cigarette smoking. • NO use of wood burning stoves. • NO use of fireplaces; frequent dusting of rooms; optional use of air cleaner.

Preventing stomach reflux	Food and stomach acids irritate throat, nasal, and eustachian tube linings.	All day, every day.	Child to sit up while eating; avoid sleeping or napping within 60 to 90 minutes of eating to permit stomach emptying; allow child to fall asleep in a swing or car seat; use blocks to elevate the head of the crib or bed or use foam, pillows to elevate the head of the mattress.
Consider and treat allergies	Many children react to airborne allergens such as pollens, dust, molds with sneezing, nasal congestion, nasal drainage. Some have food allergies.	Avoidance of exposure to airborne agents or foods. For treatment, use medications: antihistamines, decongestants, topical nasal steroids.	• NO cigarette smoking. • NO use of wood burning stoves. • NO use of fireplaces; frequent dusting of rooms; optional use of air cleaner.

DECONGESTION

Decongestion is the second arm of my ventilation routine, and it is critically important for children with persisting otitis media. My decongestion recipe for children with persistent otitis media adds "industrial strength" ingredients to mount an effective challenge against the well-established swelling of Michele's middle ear and nasal linings.

Systemic steroid pulse – antibiotic combination therapy:
The goal of this comprehensive decongestion and middle ear ventilation recipe is to drive shrinkage of Michele's middle ear, eustachian tube, and nasal linings in order to allow air to freely pass from her nasopharynx up her tube and into the far reaches of her middle ear spaces. The centerpiece of the program is the use of a short course of a systemic corticosteroid, usually *prednisolone*. Doctors call this use of the medication a steroid pulse, and the term "systemic" refers to the fact that the medication is given by mouth and is distributed to all parts of the body.

I prescribe the prednisolone, available in liquid form as *Orapred* or the generic form, in combination with a very capable antibiotic. This combination therapy eradicates resident bacteria and any frank infection at the same time that it reduces swelling of the middle ear linings. This familiar formula for success addresses the vicious cycle that swelling and ventilation obstruction induce infection and infection, in turn, induces middle ear lining swelling.

The original investigations of antibiotic/systemic corticosteroid combo therapy focused on its use for clearing middle ear fluid uncomplicated by persistent infection. These studies demonstrated that the steroid pulse was more likely to eradicate middle ear fluid, reventilate the middle ear space, and normalize middle ear pressures if it was administered in combination with an antibiotic from the mild or moderate class of antibiotics. My discussion of the various antibiotic classes may be found in the **Appendix**.

Recent studies help to explain the success of this combo therapy. Middle ear inflammation is a by-product of the bacterial release of enzymes as well as the consequence of other factors such as allergy. This inflammation from all causes is associated with a more rapid absorption of gases such as oxygen from the middle ear space and, a consequence, the more rapid reduction of middle ear pressure. The antibiotic will reduce or eliminate colonizing bacteria and the systemic steroid will reduce the inflammatory process due to all causes.

Whenever I mention the word steroid, parents typically become apprehensive. First, many confuse this type of steroid, a corticosteroid, with anabolic steroids, the type illegally used by body builders and athletes to "bulk up" and artificially energize their bodies. These two classes of steroids are worlds apart.

It is true that corticosteroids, the type I prescribe, are powerful medications with many effects as well as possible side effects, but my experience has shown that the benefits of the steroid pulse far outweigh its risks. The positives: the corticosteroid rapidly shrinks the linings of the middle ear spaces, of the adjacent mastoid cavities, of the eustachian tubes, of the nasopharynx, and of the nasal cavities. What are the negatives? The major side effect is that a child feels *very* energetic, and often becomes a "whirling dervish," unwilling to nap or to sleep at night. Rarely, the steroids may produce aggressive or belligerent behavior in a child of any age. Corticosteroids may also have an irritant effect on stomach linings, and I recommend that the steroid be taken with meals. When all is said and done, I have rarely had to recommend discontinuation of the steroids due to complications of any kind. This short pulse of steroids will not adversely affect growth.

To "blow" a burst of free air into the middle ear spaces, I recommend a relatively short 5-day pulse of the steroid. This is sufficient to produce positive changes without suppressing the function of the adrenal glands and reducing a child's own internal production of corticosteroids. If steroids are administered for 10 or more days, this type of suppression does occur, and the drug must be slowly tapered in order to allow the adrenals to resume their own steroid production.

My recipe for a cycle of antibiotic/systemic corticosteroid combo therapy directs a child to begin the antibiotic and the steroid together, to take the steroid for 5 days, to take a complete, usually 10 day course of antibiotic, and to return to see me after 30 to 40 days. This is a reasonable interval as it takes time for air to reenter the middle ear spaces following the treatment. It is a short enough interval to permit close surveillance of infection eradication as determined by a reduction in eardrum redness and swelling and by the clearance of pus from a child's middle ear spaces.

Topical steroid nasal instillation:
Michele has swollen nasal linings that extend from the front of her nasal cavities back into her nasopharynx, the name of the upper throat where the throat meets the nose and where her eustachian tube openings scoop up air to pass it up into her middle ear spaces. Extreme ventilation of the nasal cavities requires the addition of a topical nasal steroid to the recipe.

Topical nasal corticosteroids, the most popular ones approved for use in children being *Nasonex*, *Flonase*, and *Veramyst*, are medications typically used for the control of nasal allergies. They are administered once or twice a day and lead to long-term shrinkage of tissues.

Again, the questions about steroid use arise, particularly since these agents are used for weeks to months. By directly applying the corticosteroids on the nasal linings, smaller amounts of the drug may be used. To create the same concentration of the same medication in the nasal tissues, a significantly greater amount of drug would need to be introduced into the body by the oral route.

In addition, this latest generation of topical nasal steroid sprays includes agents that have been fine tuned to minimize effects on tissues other than their intended targets. The corticosteroids contained in these sprays are rapidly converted to metabolically inactive agents once they reach the circulation. Long-term studies of children who have received topical corticosteroids, usually via inhalation for reactive airway disease and bronchial asthma, indicate that these medications do not adversely affect linear growth over time.

Despite these reassuring facts, I attempt to minimize the intensity and duration of treatment with topical nasal steroids. Some children are more sensitive to these medications or absorb more of them. As a result, parents of such children occasionally report that their children experience disrupted sleep if the spray is given in the evening or before bedtime. Moving the spray to an earlier time or changing the medication often helps. Other children experience nasal lining irritation and some nosebleeds after using these agents for extended periods. Application of over-the-counter antibiotic ointments such as generic triple antibiotic ointment, *Neosporin*, *Polysporin*, or *bacitracin* on the linings just inside the nose using cotton applicators such as Q-tips will effectively prevent such irritation and heal the linings.

Prior to spraying in the topical steroid, the nasal linings should be cleansed with a spray of saline in order for the steroid to properly absorb through the linings. The cleansing removes mucus from the surface of the nasal and throat lining prior to application of the medication. Saline mist nasal irrigations of this sort should be used prior to instilling any topical nasal medication.

Because many children like Michele have excessive nasal lining swelling, the topical nasal steroids have difficulty penetrating back into each nasal cavity and into the upper reaches of each nasal cavity. Initiation of therapy becomes a "boot strap" operation.

To promote better initial penetration of the topical steroids, I recommend use of a topical nasal decongestant such as *Little Noses Decongestant Drops* for infants, *Mild Neo-Synephrine nasal spray* for younger children, and *Afrin* spray for older children and adolescents. The Little Noses and Neo-Synephrine both contain the drug *phenylephrine*, a first cousin to the natural decongestant adrenalin. The *Afrin* contains a similar but more powerful and longer-acting medication, *oxymetazoline*. All three nasal sprays rapidly shrink the nasal linings by sending the lining's blood vessels into spasm. This rapid shrinkage then allows the steroid spray that follows to reach more of the nasal linings further back in the nose. When using this nasal decongestant-steroid combo, first instill the saline mist, then spray the topical nasal decongestant, wait 10 minutes to allow for the "flash" shrinkage of the nasal linings, and then spray in the topical nasal steroid.

I usually recommend an initial 3 to 4 week course of the topical nasal steroids for children of all ages. For infants and toddlers with relatively short nasal cavities and linings with less "wear and tear," this treatment is sufficient. For older children, depending upon their initial response, I may suggest continuation for another 4 to 6 weeks with a taper of the medication at its conclusion.

Typically, the steroid nasal spray initially shrinks the linings in the front of the nose, while the linings in the back of the nose take longer to respond. After the maximal effect is reached with all nasal lining swelling resolved, the topical nasal steroid medication is stopped. It may be subsequently restarted for recurrence of nasal congestion or its persistence following a "cold."

Saline mist irrigations:
Use saline mist nasal irrigation daily and prior to instillation of any topical medicated nasal sprays such as topical nasal decongestants and/or topical nasal steroids. Do this as often as possible with a minimum administration frequency of 3 times a day. During "colds" or significant nasal congestion, double the frequency of administration to 6 times a day.

Oral decongestants:
Topical steroids are relatively weak decongestants when acute problems such as "colds" and high doses of inhalant allergens are present. At those times, for more vigorous decongestion, add specific decongestant medications. For infants and children who can only ingest liquid forms of medication, I recommend *Sudafed Children's Nasal Decongestant* which contains the chemical *pseudoephedrine*. Be forewarned that this product is not available on the pharmacy shelves, and it must be obtained from the pharmacist after showing ID, usually your driver's license. The Sudafed that you find on the shelves is *Sudafed PE*, which contains *phenylephrine*, an inferior decongestant and one with cardiac toxicity at doses appropriate for decongestion.

The strategy for administering any decongestant begins with one dose before bedtime. Your child's natural decongestion is reduced at night, and the medications your provide take up the slack. If the single bedtime dose is insufficient to control symptoms, add additional doses up to three during the day.

Older children and adolescents may use longer-acting versions of *Sudafed* such as the twice daily 120 mg extended release tablet or *Sudafed* compounded with *Claritin* or *Zyrtec* as *Claritin D* or *Zyrtec D* respectively. These are taken once at night or twice daily.

Topical decongestants:
I previously discussed the use of these medications for treatment of "colds" and allergies as well as to help initial distribution of topical nasal steroids. They are also useful for general

decongestion. Use *Little Noses Decongestant Drops* for infants, *mild Neo-Synephrine Nasal Spray* for older toddlers and young children, and regular *Afrin* for children, adolescents, and adults 6 years of age or older.

Table:
Decongestion Recipe for Persistent Otitis Media

Step	Rationale	Use	Ingredient/ Measure
Systemic Steroid Pulse – Antibiotic Combination Therapy	Corticosteroid pulse "flash" shrinks middle ear, eustachian tube, nasal, sinus linings; antibiotic eradicates persistent infection.	5 day course of prednisolone in conjunction with stronger/ strongest* antibiotics	Orapred; antibiotic selection from among the moderate/stronger/ strongest antibiotic groups.*
Topical Steroid Nasal Instillation	Use of topical nasal spray following saline mist nasal irrigation for weeks to months	Third generation topical nasal spray	Nasonex, Flonase, Veramyst.
Saline mist nasal irrigation	Moisturization of linings and mucus, cleansing away contaminants	2 sprays in each nostril 3 times a day; more often during "colds."	Simply Saline, Ocean, or Little Noses Aerosol; pump versions of Ocean, Ayr, Salinex, generic no-name saline preferred to squeeze bottles.

Oral Decongestant Compounds	Acute shrinkage and some drying of nasal linings.	Short acting agents → 2 to 4 doses/day.	*Infants*: Sudafed Children's Nasal Decongestant. *Children*: Sudafed Children's Nasal Decongestant.
Oral Anti-inflammatory Compounds	Suppresses inflammatory reactions in the nasal cavities, ear, and throat reducing nasal congestion, nasal secretions, sneezing, and cough.	Medication in liquid, chewable, and tablet form for administration 3 times a day.	Generic ibuprofen, Advil, Motrin in liquid, chewable, and tablet form.
Topical Decongestants	Powerful acute shrinkage and drying of nasal linings.	**Short acting agents:** 3 to 4 doses/day. **Long acting agent:** Twice a day. *Note*: Always administer saline mist nasal irrigation prior to a medicated nasal spray.	*Infants:* **Short Acting:** Little Noses Decongestant Drops (1/8% phenylephrine) *Older Infants and Children*: Mild Neo-Synephrine Nasal spray (1/4% phenylephrine) *Older Children and Adolescents*: **Longer acting:** Afrin (0.05 % oxymetazoline).

* Appendix

INFECTION PROCESSING

In contrast to the infection prevention strategy used for recurrent otitis media problems, eradicating the organisms associated with persistent otitis media requires a far more powerful infection processing. Michele's persistent infection continues despite use of high-powered antibiotics. When this occurs, a bacterium or a group of bacteria, resistant to many antibiotics, may be the culprit(s). One very common offender recently has been *streptococcus pneumoniae* or *pneumo* for short. Antibiotic-resistant forms of this bacterium have been floating around day care centers for a number of years. The two other possible culprits are the two other most common bacteria to cause difficult-to-treat ear infections, members of the ear infection bacterium hall of shame, *hemophilus influenza and moraxella catarrhalis*, *m-cat and h-flu* for short. These "bugs" can all develop an enzyme named *beta lactamase*, which, in turn, can inactivate many of the common antibiotics.

Add to the antibiotic resistance problem the issue of **biofilms**. These are layers of mucus that line the middle ear and eustachian tubes and encase bacteria, thereby holding these "bugs" in a form of suspended animation cavities. We are just in the early stages of understanding how to destroy biofilms and prevent them from reforming.

Eradicate persistent infection with the most capable antibiotics:

Michele has an impressive history of escalating ear infection problems. She will require an extremely competent antibiotic in order to eradicate her current infection which has already been treated with one of the most effective antibiotics available, *Augmentin ES* or extra strength. In order to obtain data to guide our antibiotic choice, I culture the discolored material I note in her upper throat, her nasopharynx, using a mini-tip culture unit. The culture report reveals her upper throat, and, by proxy, her ear, is colonized with *streptococcus pneumoniae*. It is resistant to many antibiotics including those she has been previously prescribed.

I move up the scale of antibiotic strength and recommend antibiotic therapy with *clindamycin*, one of the best oral anti-pneumococcal antibiotics and one to which Michele's *pneumococcus* is sensitive. Beyond this, we would move on to another commonly used antibiotic *ceftriaxone* or *Rocephin*, but this requires intramuscular injection therapy. For a chart listing the relative functional capabilities of commonly used antibiotics, see the **Appendix**.

This recipe should be effective for Michele, but the regimen for each child is highly variable. For the toughest cases such as this, I will recommend that the child take a full therapeutic dose of the strongest or stronger class antibiotics for two and occasionally even for three weeks. I will then reexamine the child after that time. For other infants, toddlers and younger children with less significant infections, I will follow a shorter course of a strongest/stronger class antibiotic with a consolidating course of a stronger class antibiotic to be used until the child's follow up visit with me.

If, at the follow up visit, there are signs of improvement but evidence that fluid and/or signs of inflammation are persisting, I will prescribe a continuing course of a stronger or cleanup antibiotic for another 2 to 3 weeks to permit continuing resolution of the pathologic changes. If the child's examination reveals no improvement or progression of the disease process, I will then recommend a transition to a surgical strategy.

Avoid sources of infection:
For children with persistent ear infections undergoing treatment, remaining healthy versus developing an upper respiratory infection can spell the difference between success and failure for medical therapy and sometimes for surgical therapy as well. One key to infection prevention is avoiding those people and places where infections "live." Michele is not in day care, but she

periodically attends play groups. Given her situation, I recommend that she avoid close play other children, particularly those with "green, runny noses" until she is out of the woods.

To reduce the chances of hand-to-hand followed by hand-to-mouth spread of contaminated mucus, I recommend that Michele wash her hands often, at least once for every two hours of play. As pacifiers tend to help spread infection child-to-child and may promote middle ear negative pressures and the formation of fluid, I recommend stopping or at least minimizing their use to at-home and before sleep. The verdict on whether anti-bacterial soaps and cleansers help or harm efforts to stop the spread of illness among children is not yet in. Many scientists believe that good old fashioned soap and water are the most effective and that anti-bacterial ingredients add little and may even lead to the development of bacterial resistance.

For children responding poorly to medical therapy who are in day care, I suggest a temporary change in their care situation until the crisis has passed. Care modification may include moving the child from a center day care into a home day care situation with 5 or fewer children, providing care on a temporary basis with a sitter in the child's home, or having one parent remain home with the child. The child with persistent otitis media should also avoid unnecessary contact with siblings who are ill.

Boost Your Child's Immunity:
All immunizations should be up to date, especially vaccination against *pneumococcal* bacteria, *hemophilus influenza*, and the viruses driving the "flu." Breast feeding helps to boost an infant's immune system. Unfortunately, by the time a child is identified with persistent otitis media, the decision to continue or to stop breast feeding has already been made. If you are breast feeding, know that continuing to do so will help your baby to better health.

Prevent New Bacterial Infections with Continuous Antibiotic Prophylaxis and Maximal Nasal Decongestion:
Despite everyone's best effort at helping a child such as Michele "dodge" viruses, she may develop a "cold" or other upper respiratory infection. Although she is taking a course of continuous antibiotic prophylaxis that should prevent the development of a new bacterial infection, she will employ my maximal nasal decongestion recipe to maximally ventilate her nasal cavities and middle ear spaces.

Table:

Infection Processing Recipe for Persistent Otitis Media

Step	Rationale	Use	Ingredient/Measure
Eradicate Persistent Infection	Use of **strongest / stronger* class antibody with systemic corticosteroid**s to eradicate acute infection, ventilate the middle ear space, and clear bacterial middle ear organisms within biofilms.	**Extended therapeutic course of stronger/ strongest antibiotic** for 10 to 14 days. Use 5-day pulse of prednisolone at initiation of antibiotic; follow initial antibiotic with a consolidation course of stronger/ strongest antibiotic as continuous antibiotic prophylaxis until follow up visit.	Stronger/strongest antibiotics such as Augmentin, Ceftin, Vantin / Augmentin ES, Levaquin, Rocephin used in combo with Orapred. Follow initial antibiotic course with continuation of same or lower level antibiotic until follow up visit.

Avoid Infection Sources: Day Care and Play Groups	Prefer day care and play group settings with few other children, well children, and infection transmission avoidance.	• Consider home care with a sitter or day care/play group with 5 or fewer children. • Infection prevention maneuvers at care site.	• Sitters or home day care. • Sick children excluded. • Use of saline mist nasal irrigation and humidification. • Frequent hand washing. • Avoidance of hand-to-hand contact. • Pacifier elimination.
Avoid Infection Sources: Siblings	Prevent siblings from transmitting upper respiratory infections.	• Isolate sibs who are ill. • Infection prevention maneuvers.	• Avoidance of hand-to-hand contact. • Frequent hand washing. • Use of saline mist nasal irrigation and humidification.
Avoid Infection Sources: Pacifiers	Eliminating pacifier use reduces ear infections 33-50%.	Pacifiers encourage sucking, swallowing, and negative middle ear pressures. Also pass "germs" from child to child.	If at all, only permit infants over 6 months to use while falling asleep, discontinue use for infants > 9 months of age

Boost Your Child's Immunity	• Immunizations to prevent ear infections cause by specific bacteria and to prevent severe viral upper respiratory infections. • Breast feeding reduces ear infections by 25%	• Anti-pneumococcal vaccine. • hemophilus influenzae vaccination. • Influenza vaccine. • Breast feeding	• Prevnar anti-pneumococci vaccine for infants. • Polysaccharide anti-pneumococci vaccine for older children and selected adolescents. • Influenza vaccine. • Breast-feed as long as possible.
Prevent New Bacterial Infections using Continuous Antibiotic Prophylaxis and Maximal Nasal Decongestion using the SCAADDS (scads) recipe	Following course of strongest/ stronger* antibiotic, use continuous prophylaxis with strongest*, stronger* or cleanup* antibiotic to prevent regrowth of middle ear and nasal bacteria which would drive reinfection.	Use of antibiotic daily at normal therapeutic doses until child's follow up visit. During intercurrent "colds," teething, nasal allergies, add maximal nasal decongestion [SADDS recipe or allergy recipe] using saline nasal irrigation, oral and topical decongestants with or without antihistamines.	Continuing use of antibiotic above first level class of agents. Saline nasal spray 3 times a day; oral antihistamine-decongestants such as Dimetapp or Triaminic, oral decongestants such as Sudafed, topical decongestants such as Mild Neo-Synephrine Nasal Spray or Afrin.

* - For antibiotic terminology, see Appendix.

Michele returns

Michele returns following her 2-week course of *clindamycin/ prednisolone* combo therapy. When Michele returns, her infection has resolved but her tympanic membranes remain thickened and she has a mix of air and fluid in her middle ear spaces. This is a good initial result, and to maintain and extend her gain, I suggest that she continue on continuous antibiotic prophylaxis with a full therapeutic dose of *cefprozil*, a moderate strength antibiotic, for another 3 to 4 weeks in order to prevent a relapse of infection. I also continue her use of the topical nasal steroids, as her nasal lining swelling is better but not completely resolved.

At her second follow up visit 3 weeks later, her tympanic membrane appearance and her middle ear ventilation as quantitated by tympanometry appear significantly improved. Her nasal linings are no longer swollen. At this point, I suggest that she stop the continuous antibiotic prophylaxis with *cefprozil* in favor of an episodic antibiotic prophylaxis with that same antibiotic. She will begin this antibiotic at the first sign of a "cold" and use my maximal nasal decongestion program. This recipe, the **SAADDS** recipe, is the same prophylaxis program used for children with recurrent otitis media.

The key to success of this program for all children is timing, but this is particularly true for children who have weathered a challenging run of persistent otitis media. As soon as the nose begins to run or become congested, Michele's parents should immediately begin her prophylactic antibiotic and crank up their use of the decongestants.

Once her "cold" symptoms begin to wane, Michele's parents will stop the oral and topical decongestants as well as the antibiotic. Since Michele has experienced a pattern of developing prolonged nasal lining swelling and "colds" frequently trigger the recurrence of this pattern, I suggest that her folks "punctuate" her decongestion therapy with a short course of the topical nasal steroids. As a rule of thumb, I recommend that Michele begin the topical nasal steroid *Nasonex* on day 7 of her "cold" and use it twice a day for 10 days. The 7-day delay before beginning the topical nasal steroids will permit her immune system to respond maximally to the "cold" virus before the topical nasal steroid instillation produces even mild local immune suppression.

I give her parents a refillable prescription for the moderate strength antibiotic, *Cefzil*. Since this antibiotic must be refrigerated and has a limited shelf life of 10 days when mixed as a liquid, I ask the pharmacist to dispense the medication in the unmixed, powdered form. This may be stored at a controlled room temperature range for weeks, months or even years. I also recommend that the pharmacist provide a bottle of pre-measured distilled water for use in preparing the suspension for use. Preparing the antibiotic is then simpler than baking a cake from Betty Crocker mix.

Most acute "cold" symptoms such as severe nasal congestion and nasal drainage wane by 5 to 7 days. On one occasion, Michele's parents call me to report that her nasal congestion was becoming prolonged, and she was experiencing discolored nasal drainage. Suspecting that bacterial organisms resistant to the prophylactic antibiotic were growing, I prescribed a "rescue" agent *Ceftin*, from the stronger antibiotic group, to eradicate this "breakthrough" infection, an early sinus infection which would quickly spread to her ears.

Michele "graduates"

As I see Michele back periodically through a 12 month period, she weathers many "colds" without the development of any otitis media episodes. With the coming of warmer weather, I suggest to her folks that we "dial down" the use of antibiotics. We modify her **VIP Program** for "colds" by eliminating the first "sniffle" use of antibiotic prophylaxis and the use of a "punctuating course of topical nasal steroids. With each cold, she continues to ramp up her use of saline and begin maximal nasal decongestion, but she uses no antibiotics or topical nasal steroids.

If her "cold" symptoms linger into the second week making it more likely that the "cold" will seed her ears or sinuses, we will begin the use of the prophylactic antibiotic. Initially, I give her parents an open prescription for the amoxicillin but later ask them to call if her "colds" fail to remain "well-behaved." Since all continues to go well, after another 4 months, I discharge her from my surveillance program.

When to Consider Surgery

If a child is experiencing persisting otitis media despite taking the antibiotics and following all of the strategies, then it is time for tympanostomy tube insertion. This is particularly true if the infection has persisted for more than 4 weeks, if a child is demonstrating signs of systemic toxicity such as fever, extreme irritability, consistent wakefulness and inability to be consoled, and if a child is unable to tolerate the antibiotics necessary to resolve the infections due to gastrointestinal complications or appetite suppression.

Persisting ear infections temporarily compromise a child's hearing and speech-language development. Hearing sensitivity and hearing fidelity are reduced, and they will not return to normal for many days to weeks after the infections subside. A formal hearing test may help assess the steady-state effect of infection on a child's hearing. If a child with repeated ear infections is experiencing obvious hearing difficulties or speech-language developmental delays, surgery offers the significant advantage of rapidly improving and stabilizing the hearing.

CHECKLIST: *The VIP Program for Persistent Otitis Media*

VENTILATION:
> *Cleansing:*
>> Saline mist irrigation
>> Humidification
>> Air cleansing
>> Stop stomach reflux
>> Identify and treat allergies
>
> *Decongestion:*
>> Systemic steroid pulse/antibiotic combination therapy
>> Topical steroid nasal instillation
>> Saline mist irrigations
>> Oral decongestants
>> Topical decongestants

INFECTION PROCESSING:
> *Eradicate persistent infection with the most capable antibiotics:*
>> Antibiotic treatment with a drug from stronger or strongest classes
>> Continuous antibiotic prophylaxis using moderate or stronger agent
>
> *Avoid infection sources:*
>> Care at home with sitter or home day care with 5 or fewer peers
>> Healthy playmates
>> Hand washing
>> Humidification
>> Pacifier elimination
>> Healthy older siblings
>> Vaccinations and immunizations up to date – Prevnar, anti-influenza
>
> *Prevent new bacterial infections:*
>> Continuous antibiotic prophylaxis
>> Episodic antibiotic prophylaxis
>> Maximal nasal decongestion using the SADD recipe

5 -- Recipes for Clearing Middle Ear Fluid

While recurring and persisting acute ear infections are characteristic of infants and toddlers, most children past the age of 30 months tend to be free of them. As children become older, however, a group of them begin to reexperience ear issues or experience them for the first time. This often occurs as children begin to attend pre-school and kindergarten. Driving the development of such ear problems are recurrent and chronic throat and nasal issues including adenoidal enlargement, chronic adenoidal infections, chronic nasal congestion from infections and allergies, and recurring sinus infections.

Middle ear infections in older children tend to be less symptomatic, both a blessing and a curse. While children at this age are not up at night in pain or excessively irritable during the day, they and we as parents and physicians may be unaware that a problem exists. Sometimes the only clues that a child's ears are unhealthy are apparent hearing losses, deterioration in speech clarity, or a balance problem.

Ear infections in older children develop the same way as in the infants and toddlers. Viruses and bacteria make their way up through the eustachian tubes during "colds" and other upper respiratory infections, and, while the child's immune system knocks out the viruses, the bacteria proliferate. Unlike the babies' situation, however, an older child's immune system is more competent and mounts a more vigorous response to bacteria invading the middle ear space. As a result, an acute infection with excessive middle ear pressure, pain, and fever never materializes. Often, though, bacteria and the child's immune system wage a standoff, with bacteria being produced as fast the immune system can kill them off. The process continues for days, weeks, or even months with the production of middle ear lining swelling, eustachian tube lining swelling, negative middle ear pressure, middle ear fluid, hearing loss, and balance problems.

Meet David

David is a personable 6 year old who loves to play the role of comedian. One of his favorite jokes was to feign a hearing loss, but when the school nurse called to tell David's parents that he flunked his pre-kindergarten hearing test, they were baffled. "David had many ear infections as an infant, but, when he blew out the candles on his second birthday cake, his ear infections blew away too!" his mom remembered. "Now we weren't totally surprised when he failed his screening hearing test for kindergarten, because he just doesn't listen. We always chalked that up to his age and ability to turn us off since he'd rather be playing Nintendo."

The school nurse's hearing screen showed that David did have a moderate hearing loss. It was present in both ears, but his hearing was worse in his left ear. She recommended that he visit his pediatrician, who found that each middle ear space was filled with fluid. At the time of his visit to the pediatrician, David had just been recovering from a "cold" and was also suffering from some late spring nasal allergies. His pediatrician treated his allergies with Claritin and invited him back for a visit toward the end of the summer. When he returned for that visit, his nose was clear but his middle ear fluid remained. By the time school was opening, fluid had been present and his hearing had been reduced for at least 3 months. He was now in my office for a consultation.

David's first visit

During my discussion with his folks, I discovered that, while David had been generally healthy, he did experience prolonged "colds" as well as allergy symptoms in the spring and fall. His pediatric record revealed many episodes of garden variety "colds" deteriorating into rhinosinusitis. At night, his chronic nasal congestion was joined by loud snoring, restless sleep, and occasional pauses in his breathing. His folks told me that he was difficult to awaken and prone to sleepiness during the day.

My exam confirmed that David continued to have fluid in each middle ear space. My tympanometry instrument, a sonar probe which detects air and measures the air pressure in the middle ear space, failed to demonstrate air in his middle ear spaces.

Looking for causes of his ear problems, I found much nasal congestion and signs of low-grade infection in each nasal cavity. The front portions of his nasal cavities were blocked by lining swelling and mucus which prevented a view of the back portions, but I suspected that he had a large growth of adenoidal tissue blocking the back of each nasal cavity as well.

His parents came to the visit expecting that David's next stop would be at the operating room. I told them that surgery with the insertion of tympanostomy tubes was one possible strategy, but I explained that we had other options, medical options, as well. They were enthusiastic about avoiding surgery.

We discussed the negatives as well. Since we were heading into the fall with the warm weather almost behind us, our chances of success with medical therapy were reduced. With David now in kindergarten, we wanted to optimize his hearing as quickly as possible. I told his folks that if we failed to see immediate progress with medical therapy, we would move forward with surgery

The VIP Program for Middle Ear Fluid

My master recipe for David employed maximal medical management to clean and decongest his nasal cavities as a first step toward re-ventilation of his ears. Air must pass up through the nose and into the eustachian tubes for middle ear ventilation and fluid elimination to take place. To this end, I recommended a **VIP** program which is similar in principle to the one I recommend for children with recurrent and persistent ear infections, but I modify and tailor it to the needs of the older child. For older children such as David with middle ear fluid and hearing loss, my program emphasizes **ventilation** since the immune systems of older children are more capable of **infection prevention**.

VENTILATION
The goal of my ventilation recipe for David is to **cleanse** and **decongest** his nasal cavities, his upper throat called the *nasopharynx*, a site where his adenoids reside adjacent to the entrances into his eustachian tubes, his eustachian tubes themselves, and finally his middle ear linings. David's **cleansing** routine consists of:

Saline mist irrigation:
I introduced David's folks to the concept of saline mist nasal irrigation. They had a few squeeze bottles of saline at home, but I encouraged them to purchase the aerosol version of nasal saline, available as *Simply Saline, Ocean, Little Noses,* and store brands. The squeeze bottle are sources of nasal infection as bacterial and other contaminants are drawn into the bottle when it relaxes after the contents are sprayed. Better than squeeze bottles but inferior to the aerosols are the pump dispensers.

I have suggested that David spray two sprays in each nostril at least three times a day. The regular use of saline mist irrigation washes away infecting organisms entering and residing in the nose, and studies have shown that its regular use reduces the incidence of viral "colds." As David has symptoms suggesting seasonal allergy, the saline irrigations will also help prevent allergic reactions by washing away inhaled allergens.

His mom asked if he should blow his nose after spraying the saline, and I cautioned against this practice either as a daily routine or during "colds." Nose blowing can blow potentially infected material up into his eustachian tubes or sinuses. I instead encourage David to inhale slowly while spraying the saline into his nostril in order to draw the mist-laden air through the entire extent of his nasal cavities and into his upper throat.

What about compliance? David is at an age where he will be intrigued by the spray canister, and he will likely relish the chance to push the button and perform his own applications. If it turns out that he is or becomes less than enthusiastic about the spraying, a small treat such as a Cheerio or M&M following each application will help to reinforce his willingness to cooperate. Most children initially resist spraying or dropping any liquids into the nose. As they realize that such instillations make their noses feel better and improve their breathing, they embrace their use. This was certainly true in David's case, since his mom told me that she was ultimately forced to take the canister away from him several times as he was constantly using the saline and quickly depleting the supply.

Humidification:
David's folks already have a humidifier, but they have traditionally used it only when David already had an active "cold." In fact, the consistent controlled humidification will actually prevent "colds" and other upper respiratory infections.

I encourage David's folks to buy an inexpensive humidity gauge and to place it in his room. They go one step further and purchase a gauge for every one of their bedrooms, and I applaud that decision. When the humidity level drops below the desired range of 40 to 45 percent, usually coincident with the activation of the home furnace during the colder weather, David's folks should turn on a humidifier in each room. They had an old cold mist humidifier, but I suggested that they purchase a warm mist model. For more about the whys and wherefores of humidifier ownership, see my chapter about *A Recipe for Air Humidification*.

Air cleansing:
Since David's nasal linings are already swollen, his folks must prevent him from breathing "dirty" air. Dad smokes cigarettes but only in the backyard or away from the home. Mom mentions that she can easily smell the smoke on dad's clothes. In addition, the family regularly uses a wood-burning stove.

I tell mom and dad that research studies demonstrate a significantly higher rate of nasal, sinus, ear, throat, and lung infections in children who are exposed regularly to smoke of all types. I recommend that dad stop smoking for not only the benefit of David and the rest of the family but also for himself. He will try. He and mom agree to stop using the wood burning stove and the fireplace. I also recommended that they should keep David out of rooms where dusting, vacuuming, woodworking, or use of strong and smelly solvents is occurring.

Identify and prevent allergies:
David's history suggests that he may have spring seasonal allergies. Often, children and adults who have seasonal allergies have linings that are unusually sensitive to not only inhaled allergens but to irritants of all types. I ask his folks to be on the lookout for evidence of nasal, eye, throat, or airway irritation as the result of exposures at home and out of doors.

Proactive treatment is allergen/irritant avoidance using a variety of strategies. Whenever possible, avoid extended periods of time outdoors in those zones known to contain allergens and irritants. Use frequent saline mist nasal irrigations for rapid cleansing of nasal surfaces to prevent an allergic reaction if exposure occurs. Leave clothes worn in the outdoors in an isolated mudroom or breezeway before entering the home proper. Once in the house, the child should be whisked to the shower or tub to wash the pollens or other irritants off the skin and out of the hair. This will prevent contamination of the child's bedroom.

Once the exposure occurs, so too will the allergic reaction unless treated. For medicinal prevention and treatment of allergic reactions including allergic rhinitis, I have developed a step program, which I will outline in the section describing David's decongestion recipe.

Table:
Cleansing Recipe for Treatment of Middle Ear Fluid

Step	Rationale	Use	Ingredient/Measure
Saline mist nasal irrigation	Moisturization of linings and mucus, cleansing away infectious agents and allergens from nasal linings, throat linings, and the adenoid surfaces.	2 sprays in each nostril 3 times a day; more often during "colds."	Saline aerosol highly recommended; alternative is a pump dispenser; brands include *Simply Saline, Ocean, Little Noses* but there are store brand aerosol units as well; avoid squeeze bottles
Humidification	Moisturization of linings and mucus to obtain humidity level of 40-45%	While sleeping and napping but as often as possible	Warm mist humidifiers: Vick's, Holmes, Honeywell, Slantfin
Air cleansing	Air contaminated with irritants and allergens leads to nasal, throat, eustachian tube, and middle ear lining swelling	All day, every day.	• NO cigarette smoking. • NO use of wood burning stoves. • NO use of fireplaces • DO frequent dusting of rooms and use air cleaners

Identify and prevent allergies	Reactions to airborne allergens such as pollens, dust, molds and food allergens create and perpetuate nasal, eustachian tube, and middle ear lining swelling.	Observe for seasonal and/or perennial nasal congestion, post-nasal drainage, and cough as well as ancillary allergy symptoms including itchy eyes, itchy or painful throat. Prevent such reactions wherever possible.	• Avoid allergen exposures outdoors and indoors. • Cleanse nasal linings using saline mist nasal irrigation before but particularly following exposures. • Leave clothes worn outdoors outside the home.

DECONGESTION

For David, whose eustachian tube dysfunction and middle ear fluid problems are driven by the swelling of his nasal linings, decongestion is "job one." Because his eustachian tube dysfunction is also the result of presumably enlarged and chronically infected adenoids, nursing these adenoids back to health will be critical to our success.

My decongestion recipe, in conjunction with the cleansing recipe just discussed, will first reduce lining swelling and then cleanse David's nasal tissues including the entrances to his eustachian tubes, the linings of his eustachian tubes proper, and his middle ear spaces. The recipe components will also shrink and clean his adenoids. By shrinking and cleansing the tissues in these zones, this recipe halts the vicious cycle whereby infection leads to swelling and swelling leads to infection.

Topical nasal steroids:
The workhorse medications for reducing nasal lining swelling, *edema* in medical jargon, are the topical nasal steroids including such medications as *Nasonex*, *Flonase*, and *Veramyst*. Other medications in this category are also effective, but the United

States Food and Drug Administration specifically approves the three that I have named for use by the youngest children.

Topical nasal steroids drive reduction of nasal lining edema by stabilizing cell membranes and preventing leakage of fluid into tissues exposed to irritants of all types as well as by specifically interfering with allergic reactions to inhaled agents. They are typically used for days, weeks, or months at a time.

The steroids contained in these sprays are powerful drugs, and, if administered by mouth in large enough doses to reach and affect nasal linings, would cause a variety of undesirable side effects including fluid retention, growth suppression, joint weakening, and cataracts. Fortunately, over many years, pharmaceutical research has pinpointed those steroid compounds which act most effectively on nasal linings when applied locally and which have the fewest effects on the remainder of the body. Although their predominant effect is localized, the newest agents are absorbed into the bloodstream to some extent by the body. They are readily deactivated in the liver, though, and, as a result, they produce minimal side effects, especially on a child's linear growth potential.

The safest medications for use in children include *mometasone*, branded as *Nasonex*, and *fluticasone*, branded as *Flonase* and *Veramyst*. *Mometasone* is routinely used in children aged 2 years and above, although it works safely and effectively during infancy. *Fluticasone* is approved for use in children 4 years and above.

For David, I recommend the nasal instillation of *Flonase* twice daily over the next month. As is the case whenever a medicated spray is used in the nose, several sprays of saline mist should precede application of the topical steroid in order to cleanse the linings and thereby improve its absorption.

Topical decongestants:

While topical nasal steroids act over time to reduce the swelling in the nasal linings, they must reach these linings in order to begin working. Unfortunately, David's nasal linings appear so swollen that it will be difficult for the topical nasal steroid spray to reach most of the surfaces beyond the front part of the nasal cavity. To "flash" shrink David's linings in order to allow the topical nasal steroids to reach all of them, we require a "boot strap" strategy.

To this end, I ask that his folks spray in a dose of a topical nasal decongestant following the saline and prior to the application of the topical nasal steroid. Topical nasal decongestants are available over-the-counter under the *Little Noses*, *Neosynephrine*, and *Afrin* brand names as well as no-name store brands and other generic varieties. These medications cause the small blood vessels feeding the nasal linings to constrict leading to very rapid shrinkage of the intranasal linings.

When I mention the use of decongestant nose spray to David's parents, they express concern about possible harmful effects of these medications such as rebound effects or nasal spray "addiction." It is true that these nasal sprays, if used repeatedly for weeks and weeks, will themselves irritate the nasal linings leading to the rebound effect, an ever more rapid swelling of the linings as the "shrinking" effect of the spray wears off. It is not true, however, that such medications are addicting. Furthermore, I reassure David's parents that, according to the latest studies, these medications may be used for as long as 3 weeks without harmful effects. That is a wide safety margin, since I typically recommend their use for treatment courses of 5 to 7 days or less.

These decongestant sprays are available in various strengths. For children 2 to 6 years of age, I suggest the use of *Mild Neo-Synephrine Nasal Spray*, which contains *phenylephrine* 1/4%. For children 6 years and older, regular *Afrin* containing *oxymetazoline* is safe, very effective, and long acting. For my youngest patients, the infants, I suggest the use of *Little Noses Decongestant Drops* that contain *phenylephrine* 1/8%.

The trick to using these topical nasal decongestant medications is patience. First spray in saline, then the topical nasal decongestant, then wait 5 to 10 minutes before application of a topical nasal steroid such as *Nasonex* or *Flonase*. This waiting period allows the nasal linings to shrink, thereby permitting deeper penetration of the nasal steroid spray that follows.

Systemic steroid pulse – antibiotic combination therapy:
After we clear their nasal passages and shrink their nasal lining, many children will have air enter their eustachian tubes, percolate up into their middle ear spaces, and displace the middle ear fluid. Unfortunately, other children have middle ear linings that are so thickened that the air, which enters the eustachian tube and passes up its length, fails to exit the tube and enter the middle ear space. As a result, their middle ear fluid accumulations remain.

In this situation, I will recommend more aggressive therapy: a regimen combining short courses of systemic corticosteroids and antibiotics. This therapy regimen has been studied and used over more than 30 years with safety but with variable effectiveness. While most studies of antibiotic/systemic corticosteroid combo therapy reveal fluid clearance rates of 30 to 60 % in children receiving these medications, the relapse rate over time has been disappointing in the absence of continuing therapy and vigilance.

In my experience, when this regimen is used as part of my unified decongestion recipe and employed along with my other recipes for lining cleansing and infection prevention, it works very effectively and the favorable outcome is prolonged. It has saved a large and growing group of infants and young children from surgery with tympanostomy tube insertion and sometimes an accompanying adenoidectomy.

The oral steroids work their magic in two ways. The steroids enter the middle ear and eustachian tube linings through the bloodstream, drive shrinkage of these linings, and thereby allow air to enter the middle ear spaces from the back of the nose. The steroids also reduce middle ear inflammation. This, in turn, reduces the ability of the middle linings to absorb middle ear gases, which tends to lower middle ear pressures and favors the reformation of fluid. Studies have shown that the simultaneous administration of systemic antibiotics with the steroids increases their effectiveness by preventing the growth and overgrowth of bacteria. These bacteria must be eliminated since they create swelling and inflammation, a drop in the middle ear air pressures, and the formation of middle ear fluid.

Typically, the oral steroid I prescribe is a liquid form of high dose prednisolone such as *Orapred* or its generic equivalent twice a day, each day, for 5 days. The older children and adolescents will take oral tablets to complete this steroid pulse therapy. I use 2 mg/kg/day for the youngest children, but reduce that dose to 1.5 or 1 mg/kg/day for older, heavier children in order to limit the total daily dose of *prednisolone* to 40 or 50 mg. At the same time, I prescribe a first line, mild antibiotic such as *amoxicillin* or *trimethoprim-sulfa* or a moderate antibiotic such as *Cefzil*, *Omnicef*, or *Zithromax*. In the youngest children, I will recommend continuation of the antibiotic in either therapeutic or varying dosages for a total of 30 days. In older children and during warmer weather in a non-allergic child, I will discontinue the continuous antibiotic prophylaxis but ask that the child briefly resume antibiotic therapy during upper respiratory infections including "colds."

This regimen successfully clears persistent middle ear fluid accumulations in more than 70% of children using it. When combined with my other recipes and regimens, most of the children remain free of fluid. During the warmer weather, children with seasonal allergies may "crash," while, during the colder seasons, a proportion of children will experience the recurrence of the middle ear fluid with "colds" or exacerbation of perennial allergic rhinitis. In all cases, careful management of upper respiratory infections and allergies will prevent and reverse middle ear effusions. In some cases, children will require re-treatment with antibiotic/systemic corticosteroid combo therapy or consideration of surgery.

Systemic corticosteroids predictably produce more short-term side effects than topical nasal steroids. Children may complain of stomach upset as these drugs do irritate stomach linings. The steroids can also produce hyperactivity, irritability, wakefulness, agitation, and even aggressive behavior in some children. These effects are reversible, and they disappear when the child completes the course of medication. Despite the many possible side effects and complications, only children rarely fail to complete the treatment course due to their inability to tolerate the medications.

Continuing antibiotic prophylaxis:
David's swollen nasal linings and adenoids act as "sponges" for bacteria. These germs "colonize" various nooks and crannies, and, while they fester in these locations, they drive continued swelling of the tissues and oppose the effects of our decongestion efforts. For this reason, I frequently recommend a course of antibiotics for children such as David at the onset of their ventilation therapy.

For many children with a history of persistent or relapsing otitis media, I will recommend the use of a continuing course of antibiotics until we have evidence that a child's middle ear linings are normalizing. I usually begin such continuous antibiotic prophylaxis using the antibiotic at full strength for 7 to 10 days, and I then reduce the strength by 50% for the duration of the course. I will recommend that the dose of antibiotic be increased back to a full therapeutic level during "colds" and periods of vigorous teething.

Control allergies:
I set up a recipe to help control David's allergy reactions. Like most of my recipes, the allergy recipe is a step program with the addition or substitution of medications only as needed. His folks are instructed to add various agents one at a time in order to

effectively control his symptoms. All ingredients in the program may be used with one another, when necessary, for an optimal effect.

As in so many of my other recipes, saline mist nasal irrigation is a basic ingredient. Saline spray washes away inhaled allergens such as pollens, dust or mold. The saline should be used before and after exposures, such as to cut grass, flowers, trees, or weeds.

If that alone is not sufficient, I next recommend the addition of a non-sedating antihistamine such as the drugs *Claritin* or *Zyrtec*, available in brand name and store brand formulations on an over-the-counter basis. Another ingredient to add for additional control via oral medications is *Singulair*, an example of a leukotriene receptor antagonist. Non-sedating antihistamines and leukotriene receptor antagonists block two separate pathways of the allergy response. The two may be used separately, but. when they are administered during the same episode of illness, the effect is quite powerful.

For additional control, topical medications are useful. The most universally effective agents are nasal steroids including *Nasonex*, *Flonase*, or *Veramyst*. If a child's nose is so congested that the topical nasal steroid spray hardly enters it, I recommend that a parent precede the topical nasal steroid spray with a topical nasal decongestant spray such as *Little Noses Decongestant Drops* for infants and toddlers, *Mild Neo-Synephrine Nasal Spray* for younger children 2 through 5 years of age, or Afrin nasal spray for children 6 years and over.

Other topical agents which may be helpful include the topical cromolyn spray, available over-the-counter as *Nasalcrom* and the topical antihistamines such as *olopatidine*, available as the prescription drug *Patanase,* and *astelizine*, available as *Astelin.* Cromolyn sodium is a topical agent that modulates allergic reactions in respiratory linings. Topical antihistamines operate locally in the same way as oral, systemic antihistamines operate throughout the body.

Control "colds" using the SADDS Recipe:
The sudden development and continuation of nasal congestion will oppose our efforts to eradicate middle ear fluid and normalize a child's ears. In older children such as David, it may be more difficult to determine when nasal congestion is due to a "cold" or to allergies. In general, "colds" arise more suddenly and demonstrate a typical natural history. Fatigue, a feverish feeling, and muscle aches accompany the onset of sneezing, nasal congestion, and nasal drainage during "colds." They do not in the case of allergic reactions. "Cold" symptoms then usually peak in 3 to 5 days and resolve within a week. Allergy symptoms are typically less intense, longer lasting, and not accompanied by general feelings of illness.

My recipe for treating "colds" begins with the liberal use of saline mist nasal irrigation and moves on with the addition of anti-inflammatory medications and, as needed, oral and topical decongestants. The anti-inflammatory drug of choice is ibuprofen as Advil, Motrin, or a store brand. This drug suppresses but does not totally eliminate the body's reaction to the virus including nasal congestion, nasal drainage, general muscle aches, and fever. Toward the middle of the "cold" cycle, days 3 through 5, nasal congestion and drainage may be severe enough to require additional decongestant medications.

A reasonable strategy is to add oral decongestants such as *Sudafed* first at night and then day and night. Some children are kept up by the oral decongestant, and thus a topical nasal decongestant such as *Mild Neo-Synephrine Nasal Spray* or *Afrin* will often be necessary.

Some children experience prolonged nasal congestion due to persistent lining swelling, even after their immune system has eliminated the virus. For these children, a "punctuating" course of topical nasal steroids following each "cold" will hasten the normalization of the nasal linings.

Table
Decongestion Recipe for Middle Ear Fluid

Step	Rationale	Use	Ingredient/Measure
Systemic Steroid Pulse – Antibiotic Combination Therapy	Corticosteroid pulse "flash" shrinks linings; antibiotic "sterilizes" linings and middle ear fluid.	5 day course of prednisolone in conjunction with systemic antibiotic	Orapred or generic prednisolone; antibiotic selection from among the mild or moderate antibiotic groups.*
Continuing Antibiotic Prophylaxis	Use continuous prophylaxis with mild/moderate antibiotic to prevent regrowth of residual bacterial middle ear organisms or those entering the nasal cavities in order to minimize lining swelling.	Daily antibiotic at therapeutic doses for 7 to 10 days, then half strength while fluid is present. During "colds" or nasal allergies, increase antibiotic dose to full strength, add nasal decongestion ["cold" recipe or allergy recipes].	Continuing use of mild/moderate class antibiotic: *mild:* amoxicillin, trimethoprim-sulfa, Pediazole; *moderate:* Cefzil, Omnicef, Zithromax, Biaxin.

Topical Nasal Steroids	Long-term shrinkage and drying of swollen and chronically infected or inflamed nasal linings. Normalizes nasal linings inflamed by viral or bacterial infections, allergies, or airborne irritants to normal.	Once to twice a day for weeks to months. Avoid initiation of therapy during the first 7 days of a "cold." *Note*: Always administer saline mist nasal irrigation prior to a medicated nasal spray.	*Older Children and Adolescents*: Flonase, Veramyst. *Infants and Younger Children:* Nasonex.
Topical Decongestants	Acute shrinkage and drying of nasal linings.	**Short acting agents:** 3 to 4 doses/day. **Long acting agent:** Twice a day. *Note*: Always administer saline mist nasal irrigation prior to a medicated nasal spray.	**Short acting***:* *Infants:* Little Noses Decongestant Drops (1/8% phenylephrine); *Older Infants and Children*: Mild Neo-Synephrine Nasal Spray (1/4% phenylephrine) **Longer acting:** *Older Children and Adolescents:* Afrin (oxymetazoline)

Control allergies	Eliminate reactions to airborne allergens such as pollens, dust, molds and food allergens which create and perpetuate nasal, eustachian tube, and middle ear lining swelling.	Use of step program with saline mist nasal irrigation, non-sedating antihistamines, leukotriene receptor antagonist, topical nasal steroids, topical nasal decongestants, topical nasal antihistamines, topical nasal cromolyn	**Allergy step program:** • Saline mist nasal irrigation • Non-sedating antihistamines: Claritin, Zyrtec. • Leukotriene receptor antagonist: Singulair • Topical nasal steroids: Nasonex, Flonase, Veramyst. • Topical nasal decongestants: Little Noses Decongestant Drops, Mild Neo-Synephrine Nasal Spray, Afrin. • Topical antihistamine: Astelin, Patanase • Topical cromolyn sodium: Nasalcrom

* Appendix summarizing antibiotic groups

INFECTION PREVENTION

David's fluid-filled middle ear spaces contain resident bacteria and his middle ear linings are coated with a film of mucus, a so-called **biofilm**, which encases bacteria and holds these "bugs" in a form of suspended animation. The bacteria in middle ear fluid and in the biofilms can begin to grow when a David's immune system becomes "distracted" during viral infections such as "colds" or during allergy attacks. This bacterial growth can produce typical acute ear infections but very often leads to more subtle problems such as lining swelling and excessive production and persistence of middle ear fluid.

In order to prevent these events, I recommend that David use an episodic antibiotic prophylaxis regimen, the **SAADD** recipe, during "colds."

Episodic antibiotic prophylaxis:
David is already on continuous antibiotic prophylaxis using lower dose, once a day administration. Once the "cold" strikes, he should increase his dosing to a therapeutic level by increasing the frequency of antibiotic use from once to twice a day. He will drop back to once a day use when his "cold" symptoms are resolving, usually in 7 days.

Sometimes, the mild or even moderate class antibiotics that I use for prophylaxis are insufficient to prevent bacterial overgrowth as the viral phase of the "cold" is resolving. The signs of this problem are the appearance or persistence of discolored nasal secretions with continuing nasal congestion and post-nasal drainage. Should this occur, I have asked David's parents to alert me so that I may order a stronger antibiotic.

Maximal nasal decongestion:
During any "cold," David's folks will also use my maximal nasal decongestion recipe, the **SAADDS** recipe. Since it is critical that David's nasal and nasopharyngeal linings remain minimally swollen in order to promote maximal ventilation of his ears, I

recommend an emphasis on the use of topical nasal decongestants such as *Mild Neo-Synephrine Nasal Spray* or Afrin. Some child do better with oral agents, and, if so, Children's Sudafed Nasal Decongestant would be used in place of the topical nasal decongestant or with it. At the conclusion of the "cold," he will use a "punctuating" course of topical nasal steroids to rapidly reduce any residual swelling of the nasal linings. This regimen is explained in detail in Chapter 6, *Recipes for Treating "Colds."*

David returns

When I see children such as David back in the office for a first follow up, a good proportion of them will have eradication of their middle ear fluid accumulations and normalized nasal linings. I assess his progress by examining his eardrums, the "windows" into his middle ear spaces, using my handheld ear microscope. As he improves, his eardrums thin, air bubbles appear within the fluid, and then all his fluid dries up and disappears. An invaluable tool for objectively and accurately assessing and documenting his progress is the tympanometer, a very sensitive sonar device that can precisely detect the presence of negative pressure and fluid in the middle ear space. Tympanometry will often detect improvement or deterioration in a child's ear ventilation status before it is visible. The data it provides permits me to accurately monitor a child's progress over time and to suggest timely therapy.

As well as therapy to normalize nasal linings, eustachian tubes, and middle ear spaces, I will usually prescribe a consolidating course of topical nasal steroids in order to drive maximal resolution of nasal swelling. Once the entire length of each nasal cavity is unobstructed, the topical nasal steroids will begin to reach the adenoids and drive their shrinkage as well. This process may require 4 to 8 weeks or more. Then, after the shrinkage of the nasal linings and adenoids has plateaued, I will recommend that David taper off the topical nasal steroids over a two week period. I will also suggest that his parents be prepared to restart them if he redevelops low-grade nasal congestion. Another effective use of the topical nasal steroids is to restart them for a 7 to 10 day period as each "cold" is waning.

David's Maintenance Regimen

Once David successfully clears his middle ear fluid or is well on his way to doing so, I modify his regimen to stop all continuous antibiotic use. At this juncture, our ability to maintain and extend his recovery will depend upon his development of subsequent bouts of upper respiratory infections.

I remind his folks to redouble their efforts to prevent upper respiratory infections. Measures include use of consistent and controlled humidification, generous use of saline mist nasal irrigation, and, whenever possible, avoidance of sick peers.

I transition him over to a program of episodic antibiotic prophylaxis, and this means that he will use an antibiotic only when and if he develops certain conditions which predispose him to develop another ear infection. These include the common "cold" or escalating nasal congestion due to allergies or breathing irritants. For infants and toddlers with David's type of middle ear fluid accumulation, episodic antibiotic prophylaxis would also be used during bouts of teething accompanied by excessive nasal drainage, congestion, or both.

I call this episodic antibiotic prophylaxis recipe the **SAADDS** (pronounced Sea-Adds) program. This acronym decodes as follows:

S:	saline
A:	episodic use of antibiotic during active "cold" symptoms
A:	anti-inflammatory agent ibuprofen as generic, Motrin, or Advil
D:	topical decongestant
D:	oral decongestant
S:	topical steroid nasal sprays (optional)

The success of this program is *timing*. Its most common use is during "colds," so, at the risk of being repetitive, let me go into more detail about that situation to explain how this works.

Our goal is to limit the length of the length of the "cold" symptoms, to tame the "cold." As soon as the nose begins to run or become congested, David's parents should *immediately* begin his prophylactic antibiotic and begin to administer the anti-inflammatory ibuprofen as Motrin, Advil or the generic equivalent. As it becomes necessary due to nasal blockage and drainage, they should crank up their use of the decongestants as discussed for the **SADD Program**, the recipe for "colds" discussed in Chapter 6.

While viruses cause "colds," the ever-present bacteria within the nasal cavities are always ready to overgrow and produce a secondary nasal, sinus, or ear infection. The prophylactic antibiotics help to slow the overgrowth of the bacteria, and the saline flushes coupled with the decongestants help to flush out the culture vats within the nasal cavities.

Since "colds" never begin at convenient times, I give his folks a refillable prescription for a mild or moderate class of antibiotic such as amoxicillin, trimethoprim-sulfa, or Cefzil. I asked them to fill the prescription and to have the antibiotic ready for a "call to action." When I prescribe an antibiotic such as amoxicillin, which must be refrigerated and which has a limited life when mixed as a liquid, I ask the pharmacist to dispense the medication in the unmixed, powder form. This may be stored at a controlled room temperature range for many months. I also recommend that the pharmacist provide pre-measured distilled water for a parent to use in reconstituting the powder for use.

To minimize the use of medications, I have instructed David's parents to stop the decongestants when his "cold" symptoms wane. On the other hand, if there are prolonged nasal symptoms beyond the 5 to 7 days which most "colds" last, I suspect an antibiotic breakthrough and will prescribe a moderate, stronger, or strongest class antibiotic as a "rescue" agent when David's parents notify me.

Table :
Roadmap of the SAADDS recipe:
Episodic Antibiotic Prophylaxis during "colds"

Day	Events	Treatment	Medication
1	Sudden development of mild congestion Clear nasal drainage	• Mild/moderate class antibiotic depress levels of bacteria in nose and throat • Nasal saline • Anti-inflammatory	• Amoxicillin, trimethoprim-sulfa, Cefzil. • Simply Saline, Ocean, Little Noses Aerosol saline mist. • Ibuprofen as Motrin, Advil or the generic equivalent 3 times a day.
2	Moderate congestion More and thicker drainage	• Continue antibiotic • More frequent nasal saline • Continue anti-inflammatory • Oral and/or topical decongestant at night	• Continue episodic antibiotic prophylaxis. • Continue saline mist nasal irrigation with aerosol saline mist. • Continue anti-inflammatory. • Children's Sudafed Nasal Decongestant and/orLittle Noses Decongestant Drops (for infants), Mild Neo-Synephrine Nasal Spray (for children 2-6 yrs), or Afrin (for those 6 yrs and above) at night.

3-4	Intense congestion Maximal drainage	• Continue antibiotic • Max nasal saline • Continue anti-inflammatory • Oral decongestant plus topical decongestant at night and during day	• Continue episodic antibiotic prophylaxis. • Continue saline mist nasal irrigation with aerosol saline mist. • Continue anti-inflammatory. • Children's Sudafed Nasal Decongestant and/or Little Noses Decongestant Drops (for infants), Mild Neo-Synephrine Nasal Spray (for children 2-6 yrs), or Afrin (for those 6 yrs and above) at night and during day.
7	Waning congestion Waning drainage	• Stop antibiotic • Stop nasal saline • Stop anti-inflammatory • Stop oral and topical decongestants	• Stop mild or moderate class antibiotic. • Stop aerosol saline. • Stop ibuprofen. • Stop Sudafed and topical decongestants
≥7	Continued congestion and/or nasal drainage	• Continue aerosol saline mist nasal irrigation • Topical nasal steroids	• Continue aerosol saline mist nasal irrigation. • Nasonex (under 4 yrs), Flonase, Veramyst (4 yrs and over).

David "graduates"

As I see David back periodically through the late winter and early spring, he weathers many "colds" without the development of any otitis media episodes. His tympanometry consistently reveals effective middle ear ventilation including normal middle ear pressures.

With the coming of warmer weather, I suggest to his folks that we back off the use of antibiotics. We modify his **VIP (Ventilation-Infection Prevention) Program** by eliminating the first "sniffle" use of antibiotic prophylaxis. With each "cold," he continues to ramp up his use of saline, begins use of anti-inflammatory medication, and begins maximal nasal decongestion; in short, he uses the **SADD recipe**, but he uses no antibiotics. If his "cold" symptoms linger into the second week making it more likely that the "cold" will drive a bacterial infection of his ears or sinuses, his folks will contact me. I, in turn, will suggest a course of a "rescue" antibiotic.

David moves through another quarter and remains free of ear issues. At this point, I discharge him from my surveillance program.

David was an "ideal" patient. His status normalized and remained that way. Often, though, children experience frequent fluctuations or prolonged deterioration of their eustachian tube function without redevelopment of middle ear fluid. When this pattern of disease is evident, I usually recommend that a child have frequent determinations of middle ear pressures using tympanometry at school, at the pediatrician's office, or at my office.

Another option is parental use of a consumer level reflexometer called the *EarCheck*. This device looks like an ear thermometer, but provides a measure of tympanic membrane normality by bouncing sound off the ear drum and measuring the result. The device shows a number 1 to 5 with one being normal and 5 indicating the definite presence of middle ear fluid.

I often tell parents that my level of concern about a child's ear disease is determined by a severity index, determined by multiplying the severity of disease by the duration of the disease. What do I mean by this? Mild or fluctuating ear problems such as negative middle ear pressures over months to years can be as troubling and sometimes even more significant in terms of interfering with a child's speech development and education than severe ear issues such as very negative middle ear pressures and middle ear effusions over a relatively short period of time such as weeks to months. Mild but persisting negative pressures may also create damage to the integrity of the tympanic membranes and the sound conducting ossicles attached to them.

Persisting or fluctuating eustachian tube function may cause significant communication issues. They they occur during the early years of life, they may affect the development of a child's auditory pathways into and through the brain making it difficult for normal processing of auditory information and spoke words to occur. Such children with so-called central auditory processing problems have difficulty hearing clearly with competing noise and often cannot recall spoken commands and instructions.

Central auditory processing issues and fluctuating hearing can be causative factors for and complicate pre-existing attention and/or learning difficulties. When middle ear disease of any severity lingers, it is time to obtain a formal hearing test in a sound proof booth in order to assess the effect of substandard middle ear pressures on a child's hearing. Testing for central auditory processing may be completed on or after a child's seventh birthday.

When to Consider Surgery

If a child's middle ear effusions fail to clear, if effusions repeatedly recur and persist for many months, or if a child experiences repeated bouts of more subtle eustachian tube dysfunction in association with difficulty hearing, attention and focus issues, auditory processing problems, and speech-language problems, it is time to consider a shift in strategy to surgery. If the presence of chronic negative pressure stretches the eardrum and produces weakened zones call retraction pockets, it is important to reaerate the ears quickly and consistently.

Eustachian tube functional fluctuation with its attendant changes in hearing sensitivity and fidelity will create a handicap for a child who is experiencing learning or attention problems in an educational setting. Muffled hearing exacerbates issues with auditory signal processing, auditory memory, and listening in situations with background noise. Eustachian tube problems will also create particular difficulties for a child with general developmental or specific speech delays including articulation problems.

A formal hearing test provides valuable information about the effect of middle ear fluid and middle ear lining thickening on a child's hearing, and the results should be an important factor in the decision to continue with medical management versus moving forward with surgery.

Surgically placed ventilation tubes prevent negative pressures and fluid from forming in a child's middle ear space, and, in so doing, stabilize a child's hearing. Every child's case is different. To better understand the indications for surgery, the operations themselves, and the care necessary following the operation itself, read my chapter *About Surgery*.

David's Fluid Clearing VIP Program at a Glance

VENTILATION:
    Cleansing:
        Saline mist irrigation
        Humidification
        Air cleansing
        Identify and prevent allergies
    Decongestion:
        Topical nasal steroids
        Topical decongestants
        Systemic corticosteroid pulse/antibiotic combination therapy
        Continuing antibiotic prophylaxis
        Control allergies
        Control "colds"

INFECTION PREVENTION:
    Episodic antibiotic prophylaxis:
        Mild or moderate class antibiotic
        Rescue" with moderate, stronger, strongest antibiotic
    Maximal nasal decongestion:
        Saline mist nasal irrigation
        Oral anti-inflammatory agent
        Systemic and/or Topical nasal decongestants
        "Punctuating" course of topical nasal steroids

6 -- Recipes for Treating "Colds"

Meet Greg
Greg's first visit
The SADD ventilation recipe for managing "colds"
Greg returns
Greg's maintenance regimen
Greg "graduates"
Greg's "Cold" Management Program at a Glance

Many parents tell me that they rarely use medications to control their children's "cold" symptoms. Their attitude is the less medication the better. They also mention that their pediatricians or family doctors rarely give them much guidance regarding medication strategies for "colds."

I agree that there are great benefits using medications in moderation. However, it is critical to intervene in a timely manner to prevent a "cold" from turning into an ear infection, a sinusitis, or a bronchitis. From a practical standpoint, if a "cold" goes uncontrolled, your baby or child is miserable for a longer period of time with a swollen, red, stuffed nose through which little air passes. In this unhealthy state, the nose and throat regions become a breeding ground for ear and sinus infections while dripping mucus down the back of the throat and driving incessant coughing as well as possible development of bronchitis or pneumonia.

With that background, let's discuss the interventions that will help you send your child's future "colds" to obedience school. To do so, let me introduce one of my patients who was suffering from industrial strength "cold" problems.

Before you read on, you are probably wondering if my recipe for children's "colds" is applicable to you as an adult as well. The answer is an unqualified YES so read on with self-interest as well as parental interest.

Meet Greg

Greg is an energetic three year old who attends center day care. Almost as soon as he began to spend his days with a large number of peers, he began to develop many "colds" and other upper respiratory infections.

The term *"cold"* is shorthand for a viral infection of the nasal linings and sinus air inlet passages. The term upper respiratory infection denotes an infection, usually viral but sometimes bacterial even from the outset, involving one or a number of sites in the head and neck including the nose, throat, voice box, and windpipe. An infection of the lungs would be considered a lower respiratory infection.

Normally, kids develop 5 to 7 "colds" during the colder weather, that is the fall through the spring. Greg was developing closer to 11 or 12 such infections or one about every 3 weeks. Where most normal "colds" resolve in 5 to 7 days, Greg's "colds" tended to drag on for more than 10 to 14 days. They often would result in ear infections, sinus infections, or both.

His parents wondered whether or not he might have allergies to plants, dust, molds, or even the family dog. He saw a pediatric allergist for a consultation, but his skin tests were all negative to the common inhaled antigens including trees, grasses, molds, dust, dust mites, and animal dander.

We have already focused upon management of recurrent and persistent ear infections. My discussion in this chapter will focus upon aggressive and effective treatment of "colds."

Greg's first visit

Greg, not surprisingly, was in the midst of a "cold" at the time of his first visit with me. His parents were treating him with Tylenol and over-the-counter cough medicine, so far without much success. His "cold" had begun just over a week before the visit, and it was showing few signs of relenting. Greg's usual very faint snoring was markedly louder and could be heard several rooms away from his bedroom. His sleep was also more restless, and he would awaken spontaneously most nights during his "colds." Toward the middle of the night and into the mornings, his coughing was remarkably persistent.

During his first visit with me, Greg's examination revealed a mix of air and fluid in each middle ear space but no signs of an ear infection. His nasal linings were very swollen, and pale yellow mucus was coating them. This same mucus was dripping down the back of his throat. His tonsils were slightly enlarged, and all of the linings of his throat appeared irritated. He had only small lymph glands in his neck.

What is a well-behaved "cold" and how do you housebreak your child's colds so that they fit that description? Keep reading as I share my recipes. By the way, I repeat that most of these approaches also work for adults, assuming that other medical problems do not preclude the use of the over-the-counter medications that I recommend.

As a prelude to outlining my recipe for managing "colds," I reviewed the natural history of the "cold beast" with Greg's parents. Let me do the same for you. At the beginning of a viral upper respiratory infection, the virus enters the body, travels through the bloodstream, and returns to the throat and nose. The nasal linings then become inflamed and irritated, and the sneezing begins. The nasal linings swell and begin to secrete more mucus than normal. The swelling produces the easily recognizable nasal congestion and blockage, while the increased secretions, called *rhinorrhea*, lead to drainage out both the front and the back of the nose. The secretions that come out the front coat the skin of the nostril and drip down on to the skin above the upper lip. These skin surfaces are not prepared to receive such infected secretions, and they become irritated and painful producing that characteristic "Rudolph, the red nosed reindeer" look.

Meanwhile, at the back of the nose, the post-nasal drainage pours down into the back of the throat leading to throat irritation. The secretions leak farther down and slip into your child's voice box, the *larynx*, and down into the windpipe, the *trachea*, as well as into other parts of the lower airway. The presence of these secretions in portions of the airway where they do not belong induces a cough, a reflex designed to clear secretions away from the restricted zones of the airway. Meanwhile, sneezing and misguided nose blowing create enough positive pressure within the nose and throat to drive these infected secretions up the eustachian tubes into the middle ear, deep into the recesses of the nasal cavities, and up the tear ducts into the eyes.

As the "cold" wears on, the nasal cavities, the middle ear spaces, and the sinus cavities all become so boggy and swamp-like that a new set problems begins to emerge. Even though the viruses are dropping like flies at the hands of your child's white cell "troopers," their reinforcements are emerging in the form of proliferating bacteria of three principal types: *streptococcus pneumoniae, hemophilus influenza,* and *moraxella catarrhalis,* nicknamed *pneumo, h-flu,* and *m-cat.* Unlike viruses, these bacteria can grow faster than your child's immune system can kill them. They grow in all of the boggy spaces within the middle ear spaces, within the nasal cavities and sinuses, and within the throat including the adenoids and tonsils producing a potpourri of infections including otitis media, rhinosinusitis, tonsillitis and adenoiditis, and bronchitis.

In a well behaved "cold," nasal blockage and secretion production are mild enough so that secondary sites such as the middle ear spaces, the sinus cavities, the throat, and the lower airways remain uncontaminated. The nasal cavities, middle ear spaces, and the sinus cavities are ventilated well enough that the mucus fails to become secondarily infected with our three nasty bacterial goblins. The sneezing, coughing, and nose blowing are minimal, so there is less spread.

The reasons that some "colds" are total outlaws and others are well behaved include the development and strength of your child's immune system, your child's natural powers of decongestion, and your child's pain threshold. Those annoying twitches, sneezing and coughing, are mild forms of pain. Those children with a higher pain threshold will be less likely to experience these symptoms, which themselves contribute to persistence and spread of the infection.

When the symptoms of a "cold" begin and the nasal membranes first become swollen and begin to drip excess mucus, the clock starts. Actually, the viruses which cause the "cold," usually *rhinoviruses* or *adenoviruses*, have been in the body for hours to days earlier, and they are tying up your child's immune system allowing bacteria, living in the throat and adenoids, to begin their own growth in preparation for later mayhem. Once these viruses circulate through the body and back into the nose and upper throat, they trigger swelling of the nasal linings and upper throat linings as well as the production of increased nasal mucus secretions. Usually the secretions are clear. Early discoloration is a sign that your child's body is pouring white cell "soldiers" into the area, but mucus discoloration after day 5 is often a signal that the bacterial "guerilla warriors" are already getting the upper hand in the battle. The pools of mucus, trapped between the swollen linings, are ideal settings for bacterial growth, and the bacterial population may double within 18 to 24 hours!

A child's immune system typically makes a vigorous reaction to the invading viruses and eliminates many of these invading germs within the first 5 days. The problem is that the body requires some help from parents in order to hasten the resolution of the viral infection and prevent it from becoming a bacterial infection. I call that first aid for "colds" my **SADD** recipe for maximal nasal decongestion, and I introduced it to Greg's parents.

The SADD recipe for managing "colds"

The key to controlling "colds" is controlling the accumulation of mucus debris and the tissue swelling associated with these viral nasal infections. At the first sign of a "cold," I suggest that parents *immediately* begin ventilation recipe steps for cleansing and decongestion in order to insure that the contamination and swelling of their child's nasal linings never progresses to the point of "no return," the point where a normally self-limited viral infection transitions to a continuing bacterial infection.

The acronym **SADD** decodes to list the components of that recipe:
S: saline mist irrigation
A: anti-inflammatory medications
D: oral decongestants
D:topical nasal decongestants

Before discussing each of the recipe's ingredients in turn, lets look at a road map of the average "cold" and the use of the various ingredients on a day-by-day basis.

Table:
Treating the well-behaved cold day by day

Day	Events	Treatment
1	**THE COLD BEGINS:** • Mild congestion • Clear nasal drainage	•**S**: nasal saline mist •**A**: anti-inflammatory (Motrin, Advil or the generic equivalents) 3 times a day •**D**: topical decongestant at night
2	• Moderate congestion • Increased and thicker drainage	•**S**: More frequent nasal saline •**A**: anti-inflammatory 3 times a day •**D**: oral/topical decongestant during the day and topical decongestant at night
3-4	**THE COLD PEAKS:** • Intense congestion • Maximal drainage	•**S**: Maximal nasal saline every several hours •**A**: anti-inflammatory 3 times a day •**D**: oral/topical decongestant during the day and night
6	• Waning congestion • Waning drainage	• Less nasal saline • Reduced decongestants
≥7	**THE COLD RESOLVES:** • Minimal congestion • No drainage	• Stop saline • Stop decongestants

Saline

Beginning during the early phases of a "cold" when nasal congestion or drainage is first noted, parents begin the more frequent of the saline sprays. Instead of instilling the saline three times daily, one to two puffs of the spray should be applied 6 times daily during the daytime to dilute and flush back nasal secretions.

After spraying saline into the nasal cavities, allow it to flow toward the back of the nose and down the throat. Resist the temptation to use a nasal suction aspirator, such as the one that was supplied in your newborn kit. DO NOT ENCOURAGE TODDLERS AND CHILDREN OF ANY AGE TO BLOW THE NOSE. Nose blowing and nasal suctioning both move more heavily contaminated mucus from the back of the nose and the adenoidal region forward into the eustachian tube openings and into the ventilation ports for the sinuses within the nose.

You cannot overuse nasal saline spray, as it is drug-free and chemically balanced to be as similar to natural secretions as possible. Some parents are such good saline sprayers and their children's nasal congestion limited enough that none of the other decongestant medications are necessary. Frequently, though, as a "cold" wears on, more decongestion is necessary. Saline also prevents the decongestant medications from producing excessive nasal dryness and crusting.

Many commercial forms of nasal saline spray have been available for years. The content of these products is usually the same: isotonic saline, which means that the concentration of the contained salt is adjusted to mimic that of natural body secretions. The main issues is the type of dispenser used to deliver the saline.

Most of the saline preparations are packaged in squeeze bottles and contain preservatives. This includes the branded products *Ocean*, *Ayr*, *Little Noses*, and the no-name generic store branded versions. The problem with this type of dispenser is that contaminated mucus or other liquids are suctioned back into the bottle when the user releases the grip.

A safer type of dispenser is the pump type bottle that has a one-way valve that prevents back flow of contaminated fluid into the bottle. To deliver the spray, the user puts a finger on either side of the nozzle and pulls the nozzle back. This works fairly well, but may be difficult to find. Also, since there may not be positive pressure within the bottle, contaminants may still find their way into the reservoir.

Even safer and my recommendation to you is the latest form of nasal saline spray: the aerosol saline spray. Several brands are packaged in this form including *Simply Saline*, *Ocean, Little Noses,* and no-name store brands. Each of these units has as its main ingredient the normal or isotonic saline, the same concentration of saline normally found in human secretions. Some of these manufacturers also produce another type of saline called hypertonic saline. This type of preparation has as its principal ingredient a more concentrated form of saline. Although some physicians recommend the hypertonic formulation as the unnaturally high concentration of the saline causes the nasal linings to shrink, I feel that the concentrated saline is irritating to the nose. Since I recommend constant use of the saline as an irrigating mist, I do not want it to be an *irritating* mist as well.

Parents ask, "How do I get my child to let me use the nasal sprays?" My answer is that, most of the time, you need only get your child to **try** the sprays. Once they do, they will usually notice an improvement in their breathing and will welcome the subsequent applications of the spray. Some children, however, hate to try the sprays or have difficulty adjusting to their use. For them, I usually recommend a post-spray reward such as a treat, edible or otherwise, or a favorite activity.

Anti-inflammatory Agents
The "work horse" medicine for management of "colds" is the over-the-counter oral anti-inflammatory agent. Most of us use these drugs after athletic injuries such as ankle sprains or back strains. They are multi-talented agents which inhibit the reactions of our tissues to injuries and to infection. They block the swelling of injured tissues and the accumulation of fluid between cells.

With this in mind, think of "colds" and other forms of rhinitis as "sprained noses" The use of the anti-inflammatory medications in these instances will reduce nasal congestion, anterior and post-nasal drainage, as well as the irritability of the nasal lining and the tendency to sneeze. They also reduce the irritability of the entire respiratory tract and the tendency to cough.

The most useful and safe anti-inflammatory agents are members of a class known as non-steroidal anti-inflammatory drugs or NSAIDs for short. Included in this family are the widely-used medications ibuprofen (*Motrin*, *Advil* or the generic equivalents) and *naproxen* (*Aleve*). Another NSAID is *aspirin*, but *ASPIRIN SHOULD NEVER BE USED IN CHILDREN* due to its association with a deadly necrotizing form of liver inflammation known as Reye's Syndrome. NSAIDs all reduce tissue inflammation by counteracting the cyclooxygenase (COX) enzyme which help to synthesize prostaglandins, important triggers of tissue swelling and increased lining secretions.

These NSAID "miracle" drugs, however are imperfect "miracles." They, like *aspirin*, can irritate stomach linings, thin the blood, and, in a select number of individuals, exacerbate asthma. For this reason, they must be used carefully, taken on a full stomach, and, in those with gastrointestinal issues, asthma, bleeding tendencies, or upcoming/recent surgery, only used with the advice and consent of your child's pediatrician.

For routine "cold" management, I recommend that ibuprofen as *Advil*, *Motrin*, or the generic equivalents be taken three times a day starting at the first signs of the upper respiratory infection and used each day for one week. I suggest ibuprofen rather than some of the other agents, as it has been in use longer for children of all agents than other NSAIDS.

Decongestants

The natural history of a "cold" is such that during its midpoint, usually days 3 through 5 and sometimes before, the anti-inflammatory ibuprofen is insufficient to completely decongest a child's nasal cavities and stop nasal secretions from creating post-nasal drainage. The use of saline mist nasal irrigation alone will thin and clear obstructing mucus from each nasal cavity, and this will often create significant relief. Although I recommend that children in day-care, pre-school, and school use the saline mist irrigations at least three times each day under normal circumstances to prevent contracting "colds," additional instillations of the saline will be necessary during a "cold."

If saline mist nasal irrigation added to the anti-inflammatory agent is insufficient to clear a child's nasal cavities, the next ingredient to add is a decongestant. Most parents feel more comfortable beginning decongestant therapy with an oral, over-the-counter decongestant. This agent triggers the blood vessels in the nose and but also elsewhere in the body to constrict. The constriction of nasal blood vessels reduces the swelling of nasal linings and slows their production of secretions.

The most common over-the-counter oral decongestant is *Sudafed*, the brand name for pseudoephedrine. For all infants and children, I recommend the use of *Children's Sudafed Nasal Decongestant*, but you will not find this product on the shelf. You must obtain the product from the pharmacist behind-the-counter using your driver's license as identification as *Sudafed* is now a controlled substance due to its use in synthesizing methamphetamine.

What are the downsides to the use of *pseudoephedrine*? Of most importance is that fact that, since the pseudoephedrine acts on *all* blood vessels, its continued use may raise your child's blood pressure. This possibility leads me to recommend moderation. Another common side effect is the so-called "adrenalin effect." Since *pseudoephedrine* is the first cousin of the natural body energizer adrenalin, it may also keep your child awake at night and create irritability during the day. Should this become an issue, topical decongestants, discussed below, are a good alternative.

What about duration of action? The available liquid and chewable versions of *Sudafed*, both brand name and no-name, are short acting, and it is often necessary to repeat doses 3 to 4 times a day. Unfortunately, at this time, there are no long-acting liquid versions of pseudoephedrine. There are long-acting caplet and capsule versions of *Sudafed* and generics for use with older children and adolescents who weigh 100 lbs or more. The twice a day 120 mg *Sudafed* is the most appropriate and preferable to the once daily 240 mg version. Remember, for older children who have a difficulty with pills otherwise appropriate for them according to their age and weight, embedding the pill in a peanut butter "glop," in a cheese ball, or even in some marshmallow fluff may permit them to swallow the medication.

What about Antihistamine-Decongestants?

For many years, the most common "cold" medicines for children were the antihistamine-decongestant compounds. The best-known medications in this group are *Dimetapp* and *Triaminic*. The medications in this class contain a first generation, potentially sedating antihistamine and a systemic decongestant. The antihistamine and the adrenalin-like decongestant neutralize each other's undesirable side effects so that children are not kept awake at night nor are they excessively drowsy if the medication is used during the day.

Several years ago, due to the reclassification of *Sudafed* as a controlled substance, these medications were reformulated. Rather than continuing to include pseudoephedrine, the most effective and safe systemic decongestant for children, and ask parents to buy it from the pharmacist directly, the manufacturers "weaseled out" and switched the decongestant to the unregulated *phenylephrine* to make it easier for parents to continue its purchase off the shelf. To make matters worse, the makers of

Sudafed continued to call the *phenylephrine*-containing product *Sudafed*, but merely tacked on the initials PE at the end.

Phenylephrine, an extremely competent and safe topical decongestant marketed under the brand name *Neosynephrine,* is less effective and less safe as a systemic agent. In order to decongest the nasal cavities, *phenylephrine* must be administered at a dose potentially dangerous to the heart and blood vessels. For this reason, the manufacturers have kept the dose of *phenylephrine* low. It is so low, that it is largely ineffective. Recognizing this fact, the United States Food and Drug Administration has deemed these *phenylephrine*-containing medications ineffective and not recommended for children 2 through 6 years. Since the risks of overdosing low weight infants with *phenylephrine* at any concentration looms large, the FDA labelled such preparations dangerous for infants and ordered infant preparations off the market. I don't recommend their use for another reason as well. Some studies have suggested that the antihistamines in them dry out mucus and thicken any middle ear fluid thereby preventing middle ear ventilation and effective nasal and sinus lining function.

Topical Decongestants
As the congestion associated with "colds" peaks on day 3 to 4, saline mist nasal irrigation as well as oral anti-inflammatories and oral decongestants may be inadequate to control nasal congestion and drainage. It is then, if not before, that you should begin industrial strength decongestion using topical nasal decongestants. Products are available in this category for infants and children of all ages. Use *Little Noses Decongestant Drops* (1/8% phenylephrine) for infants, *Mild Neo-Synephrine Nasal Spray* (1/4% phenylephrine) for toddlers or children younger than 6 years, and *Afrin Original Spray* (0.05% oxymetazoline) for children and teens 6 years or older including adolescents and adults.

Topical nasal decongestants may be used along with systemic decongestants or in place of them particularly at night since they do not keep children awake. They should be administered about 15 minutes before bedtime to allow the medication to shrink the linings and open the nasal airway before the child gets in the crib or bed and lays down. Head down postures always exacerbate nasal congestion. *Little Noses Decongestant Drops* and *Mild Neo-Synephrine Nasal Spray*, the agents used for the infants and younger children, have a 4-hour duration of action. Afrin, on the other hand, has a stated 12-hour duration of action but, in reality, an 8-hour duration of action. For that reason, it is often necessary to repeat the *Mild Neo-Synephrine Nasal Spray* and *Little Noses Decongestant Drops* with at least one additional dose at night.

To improve the absorption of topical nasal decongestants, I advise that parents first use saline mist nasal irrigation to cleanse the surfaces of the nasal linings. If a child's nasal linings are very swollen and the child's nose is totally blocked, it is often necessary to use two sequential doses of topical decongestant medication in each nasal cavity. Space the doses 5-10 minutes apart to permit the maximal effect of the first dose to "pave the way" for the second dose.

Topical decongestants may be used together with oral decongestants and anti-inflammatory agents. They work as a team. At the peak of a "cold," it is very possible that a child may be using three to four doses of both topical nasal decongestants *and* topical decongestants or antihistamine-decongestants.

Periodically, parents may mention that their child seems jittery or nervous when taking these products. If that occurs, I would back off on the oral medication and use the more effective but not absorbed topical form.

Humidification
Nasal and throat linings swell more readily when they are dry. Even when a child is healthy, I suggest consistent use of a

humidifier to maintain the relative humidity in a child's room between 40 to 50%. This is critical in order to maintain sufficiently moist and healthy linings in the nose, throat, eustachian tubes, and, most importantly, in the middle ear. The need for humidification intensifies when a child has a "cold."

During "colds," the additional humidification is extremely useful as an adjunct to the saline mist nasal irrigation. I suggest raising the relative humidity an additional 5%, to a level of 45 to 50%, which helps to maintain the fluidity of the mucus layer in the nose, eustachian tubes, and sinuses. This extra moisturization also helps the saline mist nasal irrigations counteract the drying effects of the decongestant medications.

I recommend the use of a **warm mist humidifier** such as models manufactured by Honeywell, Holmes, or Vicks. It turns out that most of the warm mist humidifiers are manufactured by Kaz Industries under the various brand names. Look for a model with more than a 2-gallon capacity, a built-in humidistat that controls the vapor production to keep the room's humidity within the moderate range, and, ideally, an internal fan to mix the pure water vapor with room air in order to cool it and distribute the humidified air around the room. I will tell you more about humidifiers in the chapter *A Recipe for Air Humidification*.

Cooking Up A Storm

The creative part of parental "cooking" is learning to use these medications together in order to play your child's "cold" like a virtuoso. Don't take a wait and see" attitude when you first spot the beginning of "cold" symptoms. *Immediately* begin to use more saline mist nasal irrigation and begin the use of anti-inflammatory medication. Then, be prepared to first increase and then reduce the use of the decongestant medications, both oral and topical, as your child's symptoms wax and wane. Be creative and experiment! You know your child best, and *you* can call the shots better than the professionals sitting miles away in their offices.

Antibiotics -- Friends or Foes?

What about antibiotics? Most infants and children without ear infection or sinusitis problems do not require the routine use of antibiotics during "colds." Viruses cause "colds," and antibiotics will not prevent "colds" from occurring or treat the viral infection itself. Your child's body makes a vigorous immune response to viruses, and the immune system is able to eliminate most "cold" viruses and the primary illnesses they cause within 5 to 7 days of their onset.

Unfortunately, some "colds" drag on beyond the point where a child's immune response should have overcome the viruses that initiated it. The most common reason for sustained "cold" symptoms is continued nasal and sinus lining swelling due to a lack of cleansing and decongestion. When nasal linings remain swollen and nasal mucus sludges, bacteria begin to grow, and it is those bacteria that prolong the nasal infection. It is this bacterial growth and overgrowth that fuels the development of sinus and ear infections.

How can you read your child's "cold?" How can you determine if a "cold" is resolving or lingering? To do so, you must consider two factors: the level of nasal congestion; and the quality and quantity of nasal mucus. Determine the severity of your child's nasal congestion by your estimate of his or hear nasal airflow and by the amount of decongestant medication you must use to keep the nasal linings open. Congestion and need for decongestants typically peaks at day 3 to 4 after the "cold" begins. If the congestion is continuing to escalate beyond this point and if it is not waning by day 5 to 7, think bacterial infection.

Mucus flow and color are tougher to read. Typically, nasal drainage is clear during most days of "colds." You will see milky or discolored drainage during the first few days of a "cold" as the viruses elicit a vigorous immune response and the body's white cells pour into the nasal secretions. Discolored drainage will also occur early in the life of a "cold" if the nasal secretions are permitted to dry up due to poor humidification of room air or inadequate use of saline mist nasal irrigations. If discolored mucus appears or reappears after day 5 to 7, think bacterial infection.

Rescue antibiotics
Some "colds" are "bad actors" from their onset. Treating the badly behaved "cold" requires more aggressive therapy with more saline mist nasal irrigation and more decongestants at earlier stages in the "cold." It may also ultimately require the use of antibiotics, which I call "rescue" antibiotics.

For infants and children with prolonged congestion and discolored mucus at 7 to 10 days following the beginning of a "cold," signs which suggest the development of a bacterial infection in their nasal cavities and sinuses, I prescribe a "rescue" antibiotic. The bacteria that frequently colonize the nasal cavities of infants and children, particularly those in day care situations, are usually the same nasty agents that cause otitis media and rhinosinusitis. For this reason, I prescribe very competent beta lactamase resistant antibiotics capable of eradicating the common offending bacteria: *streptococcus pneumonia* better known as *pneumococcus*, *hemophilus influenza*, and *moraxella catarrhalis*.

Since swelling breeds infection and infection breeds swelling, the proper treatment of the nasal infection requires both maximal nasal decongestion and the rescue antibiotic. Because the most capable decongestants are topical nasal decongestants, I recommend *Little Noses Decongestant Drops*, *Mild Neo-Synephrine Nasal Spray*, or *Afrin Nasal Spray* depending upon the age of the child. Antibiotics alone will not eradicate the nasal or sinus infections and the ear infections they promote. Nasal lining swelling creates a "swamp" environment that favors persistence and relapse of infection.

The mechanics of arranging antibiotic coverage vary. I instruct all parents to put up a red flag if it appears that the "cold" is not resolving toward the conclusion of its first week. For some children, I will ask parents to call me, discuss the situation, and I then call in a script for the antibiotic. For others, I provide a "security script," a standing, refillable script which mom and dad may use when a "cold" appears to be escaping control. To facilitate the timely use of antibiotics, I often ask the family's pharmacist to dispense the antibiotic in the unreconstituted form, as powder, and I also ask the pharmacist to provide a second bottle with a measured volume of distilled water. This permits mom or dad to easily and safely prepare the antibiotic for use by merely pouring the distilled water slowly into the bottle of powder in order to reconstitute the liquid antibiotic.

The table below demonstrates the type of therapy necessary for a poorly behaved "cold."

Table:
Treating the poorly-behaved cold day by day

Day	Events	Treatment
1	• Congestion • Clear to cloudy nasal drainage	• Nasal saline every 2-4 hours • Anti-inflammatory oral agent - ibuprofen • Oral decongestant - Sudafed
2	• Intense congestion • More and thicker drainage	• More frequent nasal saline • More frequent anti-inflammatory oral agents • More frequent oral decongestants • Topical decongestants - Little Noses Decongestant Drops, Mild Neo-Synephrine Nasal Spray, Afrin nasal spray
3-4	• Intense congestion • Thicker drainage	• Maximal nasal saline • Maximal anti-inflammatory oral agents • Maximal oral decongestants • Maximal topical decongestants
6	• Intense congestion • Discolored drainage	• **Consider "rescue" antibiotic** • Maximal nasal saline • Maximal oral decongestants • Maximal topical decongestants
≥7	• Intense congestion • Discolored drainage Cough	• **"Rescue" antibiotic** • Maximal nasal saline • Maximal oral decongestants • Maximal topical decongestant

Prophylactic antibiotics

For children who have an established history, that is a long "rap sheet" of ear or sinus infections occurring in association or following each "cold," I recommend the use of immediate episodic antibiotic prophylaxis at the first sign of a "cold" and episodes of escalating and continuing nasal congestion and drainage. These antibiotics eliminate colonizing bacteria within the nasal cavities, within the sinuses, and colonizing the upper throat or nasopharynx even as the virus is triggering the "cold" itself and the body's immune system is eradicating the virus. With the bacteria gone or in small numbers, the viral "cold" resolves without triggering the secondary bacterial infections.

This concept continues to be confusing to physicians and parents alike. We are all indoctrinated with the concept that, since viruses cause "colds," these infections should not be treated with antibiotics. Unfortunately, our nasal and throat passages host vast communities of microorganisms that influence the outcome of any acute infection. As viruses wreak havoc creating the "cold," the resident bacteria merrily grow and overwhelm the system. The prophylactic antibiotics' role is not to eradicate the viruses but rather to eliminate or at least reduce the numbers of bacteria residing within the nose, in the upper throat including the adenoids, and in the tissues at the entrances of the eustachian tubes.

In order for this program to work effectively, the antibiotic administration must be started at the very outset of the "cold." The bacteria in the nose, sinuses, and throat grow rapidly while the viruses are at play, and it is a race to get the antibiotics in place fast enough to prevent overwhelming bacterial growth. As the "cold" symptoms wane after 5 to 7 days, the antibiotics may be stopped because the "danger" is over by then.

This concept of only using antibiotics during the tenure of the "cold" is also confusing. We all expect that antibiotics must be used for 10 days, or, more recently, 5 days to one week for some antibiotics. Remember, in this prophylactic antibiotic recipe, we are using antibiotics to prevent rather than treat infection, and once the threat has passed, the antibiotic may be stopped.

I prefer to use the mildest antibiotics for use as prophylactic antibiotics. For a review of my list of antibiotic classes, see the **Appendix**. Such antibiotics, coupled with effective nasal decongestion, will prevent viral "colds" from spawning secondary bacterial infections.

Sometimes, the first line and milder antibiotics that we use for prophylaxis are insufficient to prevent bacterial overgrowth. This may be particularly true in day care attendees who tend to contract particularly resistant forms of bacteria from their peers. The signs of this problem are persistence of discolored nasal secretions and continuing nasal congestion with post-nasal drainage. This "technicolor" mucus indicates bacterial overgrowth in the nasal cavities and sinuses.

When this type of "breakthrough infection" occurs, I treat the child with a rescue course of antibiotics, chosen from my list of moderate, stronger, or strongest antibiotics. In many cases, I obtain a culture of the debris within the child's nasal cavities and nasopharynx, the upper throat, to help guide the choice of antibiotic. If this type of breakthrough occurs repeatedly, I will then strengthen the antibiotic agent used for episodic antibiotic prophylaxis during future "colds."

Another problem is the "lingering cold." After the viral infection has passed and the threat of bacterial infection is over, some children just naturally experience prolonged nasal congestion without any evidence of ongoing bacterial infection. Even in the absence of allergy, which is a possible reason for this problem, the tissue damage caused by the virus resolves so slowly that it puts the child at risk for a subsequent, late bacterial infection. To help the nasal linings return to normal more quickly in such cases, I recommend what I call "punctuating" courses of topical nasal steroids following each "cold."

I recommend beginning the use of topical nasal steroids for this purpose as the viral infection is waning, on day 7, and continuing their use for 7 to 14 days. I don't recommend the use of topical nasal steroids before day 7 of a "cold" for two reasons. The first is that topical nasal steroids are relatively weak decongestants, and, during the early phases of a "cold," it is necessary to use stronger oral and topical decongestants. The second reason, of more importance, is that recent studies suggest that topical nasal steroids induce a local reduction in immunity. Patients using these medications during an active "cold" shed virus for a longer period of time than average.

Table:

Preventing "cold" - associated ear and sinus infections

Day	Events	Treatment
1	• Mild congestion • Clear nasal drainage	• **BEGIN prophylactic antibiotic** • Nasal saline • Oral anti-inflammatory agent • Oral decongestant
2	• Moderate congestion • More and thicker drainage	• **Prophylactic antibiotic** • More frequent nasal saline • More anti-inflammatory agent • More oral decongestant OR • Topical decongestant
3-4	• Intense congestion • Maximal drainage	• **Prophylactic antibiotic** • Maximal nasal saline • Maximal anti-inflammatory agent • Maximal oral decongestant • Topical decongestant
5-6	• Waning congestion • Waning drainage	• **STOP prophylactic antibiotic** Reduce nasal saline stop anti-inflammatory agent • Stop decongestants • **BEGIN** "punctuating" course of topical nasal steroids (optional)
≥7	• Minimal congestion • No drainage	• Continue "punctuating" course of topical nasal steroids for a full 7 to 14 days • Nasal saline

Back-to-Back "Colds"

What should you do if your child develops back-to-back "colds?" The answer is simple: treat each "cold" with the same or greater fervor. On the other hand, if persistently discolored nasal mucus quickly arises during the early days of a second or subsequent "cold" bout, consider the possibility that your child's nasal symptoms are driven by a persisting or rapidly recurring bacterial nasal infection driven by bacteria not sensitive to the antibiotic used during the last "cold." When this situation occurs, I will often suggest a nasal or nasopharyngeal culture and prescribe a stronger antibiotic in place of the original prophylactic agent.

One more bit of wisdom about antibiotics: as Ben Franklin said, "a step in time saves nine," and the timely use of weaker antibiotics will prevent the need for longer courses of stronger antibiotics. As you know from reading newspapers and magazines, antibiotic overuse has driven the development of resistant bacteria. The publicity associated with this phenomenon has many parents running scared and avoiding *any* antibiotic use. Don't make this mistake. At the risk of being repetitive, my programs are designed to minimize your child's use of antibiotics by the *timely* administration of antibiotic "pulse" courses in order to prevent the bacterial infections which would then require the prolonged and repeated use of stronger antibiotics.

Preventing "Colds"

For "colds" as well as for most illnesses, the best treatment is effective prevention. I remind Greg's parents to keep him away from children with active "colds." The *rhinoviruses* and *adenoviruses* that commonly cause "colds" shed from the noses and throats of ill children in greatest numbers during the first 3 to 4 days of the "cold." If Greg plays with another child who shows symptoms of a "cold," he should wash his hands frequently. The water rinse rather than the soap is most effective against the "cold" viruses. Common soaps, detergents, and even germicidal hand lotions alone will not kill "cold" viruses, but the water will wash them away or at the very least dilute their numbers. Greg should also keep his fingers and toys away from his nose and mouth, since the fingers, toys, pacifiers, and any other objects which children share will transmit "cold" viruses.

I also suggest that Greg's parents make every effort to maintain a healthy environment for him whenever possible. They have a humidifier in his room, in his playroom, and they have asked his day care manager to consider purchasing humidifiers for his day care center. They have also requested that the day care center plan regular hand washing games with the children, an idea I enthusiastically applaud.

Last but not least, the regular use of aerosol saline spray once before going to play with other children, once after returning home, and once at night reduces the chances of contracting a "cold." You cannot overuse saline mist nasal irrigation!

Greg's "Cold" Management Program at a Glance

THE SADD RECIPE FOR MANAGING "COLDS"
> S: saline mist irrigation
> A: anti-inflammatory medications
> D: oral decongestants
> D: topical nasal decongestants

HUMIDIFICATION

ANTIBIOTICS
> Rescue antibiotics
> Prophylactic antibiotics

PREVENTING "COLDS"
> Avoid sick playmates
> Wash hands frequently
> Consistent and controlled humidification
> Saline mist nasal irrigation

7 – A Recipe for Air Humidification

Why do you need air humidification?
What is the ideal relative humidity?
How can you measure relative humidity?
When should you use a humidifier?
Which is the best type of humidifier?
Which brands of warm mist humidifiers are best?
What else can I do to achieve the healthiest air possible?

Why must air be humidified?

Dry air is an important contributor to upper respiratory infections. The linings of the nose and throat detest dryness! When moist, these linings form excellent barriers against invasion by viruses and bacteria. When dry, the collect all manner of debris, develop "micro-cracks" in their surfaces, and actually increase your child's chances of developing throat, nasal, and ear infections.

The nasal, sinus, and throat linings are called mucous membranes because they are all covered with a thin layer of mucus. This mucus layer rides as a conveyor belt on the micro-hair surfaces of the ciliated lining cells, and the mucus must be moist and thin in order for it to move properly and maintain its protective function. The micro-hair are the cilia which move in waves and propel the mucus in the proper direction. If that mucus cannot move due to sludging and crusting, it cannot transport surface debris including bacteria, molds, and cell debris out of the sinuses, nasal cavities, and throat recesses including the eustachian tube openings. If it dries up and cracks, it exposes the underlying cells to dryness, inflammation, and eventual infection.

Humidification of the air is particularly important in four season climates and in desert communities. In the desert, the air is already dry, and the air conditioning necessary during the summer months accentuates the drying. For the majority of us who experience four seasons, the moisture content of the air we breathe, the so-called humidity level, begins to drop precipitously when furnaces begin to heat our homes in the winter. This is particularly true in homes that have forced hot air heating systems and less so in homes with radiators heated by hot water or steam.

Once the heat comes on in the autumn, the humidity level in the average American home begins to plummet from warmer weather levels of 40% or higher to levels below 25% by the dead of winter. The average heated home is drier than the Sahara Desert, where the average humidity level hovers at 25%. While it is ideal to humidify all rooms in the home, all bedrooms should definitely be humidified.

What is the ideal relative humidity?

The nose and throat prefer a relative humidity of about 40 to 45%. Humidity of less than 35% will lead to drying out of the nasal and throat linings while humidity of greater than 60% will facilitate the growth of molds and dust mites, a distinct problem for those with perennial allergies to these common environmental agents.

How can you measure relative humidity?

It is easy to measure relative humidity within a room using an inexpensive humidity gauge, technically known as a *hygrometer*. These are available as relatively inexpensive units in combination with a thermometer and are manufactured by the Springfield and Taylor companies. They are sold for approximately $8 to $10 at most independent hardware stores, many of which are associated with the Ace or TruValue chains. Several manufacturers also produce an electronic version of the humidity and temperature gauge, sold for approximately $10-30. These units are more accurate and take measurements more quickly than the mechanical ones, but they may or may not be worth the additional expense.

When should you use a humidifier?

When the outdoor temperature drops below 40°F during the day, night, or both, it is time to turn on the humidifier. As a rule of thumb, bedroom air will require humidification when your furnace is operating.

Which is the best type of humidifier?

Five types of humidifiers are in common use today. These are the warm mist humidifier, the steam vaporizer, the cool mist humidifier, the ultrasonic humidifier, and the evaporative humidifier. I recommend the warm mist humidifier as the safest and most effective.

The **warm mist humidifier** is a safe variant of the steam vaporizer. In both, the machine boils the water and only emits steam, which is pure water vapor. Any bacteria or molds which contaminate the water in the reservoir will not be passed into the air and from there into your child's throat or lungs. This is the case since water vapor is composed of pure water molecules, not of droplets. The vapor is pure water, and none of the common airborne contaminants such as bacteria, molds, or chemicals in the water can piggyback on the vaporized water molecules.

Warm mist humidifiers in contrast to vaporizers also include a *humidistat*, a device that turns the steam generator off once the humidity in the room reaches the desired level, which is 40 to 45%. Vaporizers have no humidity controls, and they continue to produce steam that may elevate the room humidity to dangerous levels causing the proverbial clouds to form on the ceiling. Turning your child's room, or your room for that matter, into a rain forest is not healthy since molds and dust mites will proliferate.

The best warm mist humidifiers also contain a fan to completely mix the room air with the steam and to distribute the blend around the bedroom more efficiently. This mixing process also cools the steam-filled air exiting the humidifier making it less hazardous to a little hand accidentally roaming into the wrong zone. Unfortunately, cost-cutting over the past few years has removed fans from many of these units. If you have or buy a warm mist humidifier which does not have a built-in fan, buy a separate small safety fan with soft rubber blades and place it behind the humidifier so that its gust blows by the vapor outlet in order to better mix room air with the steam, cool that stream, and to better circulate the mix around the bedroom. Place the unit up on a high table or well-anchored shelf away from probing fingers.

Cool mist or ultrasonic humidifiers spray very tiny droplets of water from the reservoir tank into the air. These units are unsafe since they will spray any contaminant contained in the water within their reservoir tanks into the air and into your child's lungs. As water sits around in the tank at room temperature, bacteria and mold will grow and the water becomes contaminated. Although these units have filters, these germs as well as any chemicals in the water, will be blown around the room in micro droplets. This airborne debris also coats all walls and furnishings and is often described as "white dust." Of more importance, this material will coat the linings of your child's nasal cavities, mouth, throat, sinuses, eustachian tubes, and tracheobronchial airways.

Ultrasonic humidifiers are particularly dangerous, since the particle size they generate is smaller than that generated by a conventional cool mist humidifier. These smaller particles are better able to penetrate more deeply into the lungs and sinuses carrying contaminants into normally sterile zones. This situation may breed particularly nasty forms of pneumonia and sinusitis. Thus, ultrasonic humidifiers literally "weaponize" the contaminated water within the reservoirs.

Cool-mist or ultrasonic humidifiers must be carefully cleaned on a daily basis, an impossible task for most of us. Disinfectants and filters must be purchased and used consistently. On the other hand, steam-based warm mist humidifiers need not be cleaned as often or as carefully. While it is true that the minerals and other chemicals which remain in their heating chambers after the pure water vapor is boiled off should be periodically rinsed out and scrubbed off the heating coils or plates, even if it is not removed this residue represents no threat to your child's health. Use of soft water will prevent the mineral deposits, and some warm mist units include filters to "soften" the water. With a warm mist humidifier, the purity of the air leaving the unit is never at risk.

The **evaporative humidifier** is a common type sold to humidify larger areas of the home. They are often floor units that are designed to sit in the hallway. They may also be attached to a central heating system which uses forced hot air. They operate by passing air over and through a cloth wick that dips into a water reservoir. The wick may actually be a belt that is rotated through the reservoir. Unfortunately, the water reservoir, as was the case for cool mist and ultrasonic humidifiers, is a breeding ground for bacteria and molds. They then coat the rotating belt and are blown into the outflow channel of the humidifier and into your child's nose and throat.

Which brands of warm mist humidifiers are best?

Over the years, Honeywell, Holmes, Vick's, and Slantfin have manufactured the most reliable, cost effective, and feature-laded warm mist humidifiers. Some rather good models are also sold under the Sears brand name. The best, most cost effective unit is a moving target. For example, all of the models just mentioned are now manufactured by one company named Kaz Industries.

When purchasing, look for models with at least a 2-gallon capacity. Choose a unit with a continuous control humidistat rather than those with only high, medium, and low humidity settings. Also, some humidifiers have power controls which control the level of mist output, not the actual humidity. On such controls, the high – medium – low settings actually refer to the heating power generated by the unit, not the ultimate room humidity level you wish to reach. Some of the newest models may have electronic humidistats that permit you to dial in a relative humidity level. Some of these humidistats are capable of remote operation and some are fixed on the humidifier. If you buy a unit with a fixed gauge, check that the humidity level shown at the humidifier is that same as that near your child's bed by using a separate humidity gauge.

You should be able to purchase an effective unit in appliance stores, hardware stores, or online for anywhere from $40 to $120 depending on reservoir size and features. As always, check articles in consumer magazines and read online reviews to see the latest feedback on the latest models.

What else can I do to achieve the healthiest air possible?

Air humidification is one giant step. Add to that the elimination of all airborne smoke from wood burning stoves and fireplaces. Prohibit smoking of cigarettes, cigars, or pipes within the house, and ask smokers to wear clean clothes when they visit. If you have a particularly dusty house or live in a dusty or smog-laden zone, consider the purchase and use of an air cleaner. Again, consult consumer magazines and online reviews to find the best machines at the best prices.

8 –Recipes for Allergies

What causes allergies?
How do environmental allergies cause ear disease?
How do you diagnose the existence of nasal and throat allergies?
When is a professional allergy evaluation worthwhile?
What are the recipes for preventing allergies?
What is the recipe for treating allergies?
Meet Lawson.

In earlier chapters, I discussed the role of "colds" in the development and persistence of acute ear infections and chronic or relapsing ear problems such as middle ear fluid. I like to think of allergies as slow motion "colds" with inhaled or ingested allergens from your child's environment producing many of the same symptoms, signs, and secondary bacterial infections produced by viral-induced "colds."

What causes allergies?

When a child breathes in airborne agents such as the pollens from trees, flowers, or weeds, the particles float into all of the nooks and crannies of the upper airway system including the nasal passages, the sinus cavities, the throat, the eustachian tubes, the middle ear spaces, and the mastoid cavities. In the non-allergic child, their immune system's cellular scavengers, the macrophages, quickly eliminate these foreign particles.

In the allergy-prone child, cellular elements of the child's immune system, including those same scavenger macrophages but also a family of lymphocytes, may begin to react with the airborne particles and generate an immune response to them. Many of these white cells are in the throat, located in the adenoids and tonsils. Allergy-mediating antibodies are produced by lymphocytes after a first or previous exposure to any foreign chemical including those found on the surfaces of pollens, viruses, and bacteria. Once the body reacts to a foreign agent by producing such antibodies, this agent may then be properly termed an allergen. The allergy-mediating antibodies then circulate through the body and stand ready to catalyze the development of reactions designed to help eliminate future cohorts of such invading foreign particles from the body. These reactions are termed allergic reactions.

A similar process is responsible for the development of food allergies. Instead of airborne particles, the potential triggers are the chemicals found in the foods we buy and prepare for our children. If a child is prone to develop allergies, the immune system begins to mount a response to one or more components of foods, often proteins and very often the proteins found in dairy products. These agents react with lymphocytes located in sites throughout the digestive system, and antibodies against them are produced. Then, whenever the child ingests the food again, an allergic reaction ensues. That allergic reaction may trigger swellings of the throat and other respiratory linings.

The fact that some children are prone to develop allergies and others are not may sometimes be the luck of the draw but is usually determined by heredity. If one of your parents has experienced allergies, you and your children are more likely to develop them as well. If both parents have had allergies, their offspring are even more likely to develop them.

How do environmental allergies cause ear disease?

Allergies produce lining swelling and inflammation. When allergic reactions occur in the linings of the throat, nose, and ears, swelling of those linings occur. That swelling, in turn, blocks the flow of fresh air at normal pressures into the middle ear space and into the sinuses. From there, as you already know, it is all downhill.

When an inhaled or a food allergen contacts a lining in the throat, nose, or ears of an allergic child, a child who has already made the necessary antibodies to the allergen, certain cells in that lining, including mast cells, release allergy-mediating substances belonging to a number of chemical families. Two of the most important families are the *histamines* and the *leukotrienes*. Allergy mediating members of these two families then trigger the expansion of tiny blood vessels and the leakage of tissue fluids. Both events leading to tissue swelling as well as inflammation heralded by itching and lining redness. If the reaction is severe, so much tissue swelling and inflammation occurs that breathing passages may become dangerously narrow and so much blood vessel relaxation occurs that a child's blood pressure may drop to dangerous and life-threatening levels. This most severe form of allergy is known as *anaphylaxis*.

How do you diagnose the existence of nasal and throat allergies?

The task of diagnosing allergies is challenging, and parental observations are as effective as physician's tests. Parents should be suspicious about the existence of nasal and throat allergies when "cold" symptoms are low grade but prolonged or when mild "colds" occur one after another.

Another tip off is the occurrence of such symptoms at particular times of the year. The spring allergy season, the peak period for reactions to grasses, flowering plants, and most trees, begins in mid-April and lasts through June or beyond. The fall allergy season, the peak period for reactions to weeds, some molds, and select plants and grasses, begins in mid-August and extends into October or until the first frost. If nasal congestion seems to transcend the seasons, perennial or year-round allergies are likely. Children with perennial allergies experience reactions to the seasonal allergens as well as to allergens that remain with us throughout the year including dust, dust mites, molds, foods, and animal dander.

If you find that your child's nasal reactions occur predictably during either the spring or fall allergy seasons or during both, you can infer that your child has allergies to agents indigenous to that season or seasons. For such periodic and well-defined allergy reactions, it is possible to avoid exposure to the allergens and use medical therapy to suppress a child's reaction to it.

When is a professional allergy evaluation worthwhile?

If there is evidence of allergic reactions for more that 4 months of the year or if seasonal nasal allergic reactions are accompanied by wheezing, chronic coughing, or shortness of breath, I recommend that a child have a formal allergy evaluation and appropriate skin testing. Formal allergy evaluations are most often conducted by pediatric allergists, sub-specialists with advanced training in immunology and its application to the diagnosis and management of childhood allergic reactions. Some ear, nose, and throat specialists with special interests and advanced training in allergy and immunology may also perform such work-ups. In either case, the consultation consists of extensive history taking, a physical exam, skin testing, and, depending upon circumstances, pulmonary function testing and blood testing. Antihistamines and oral steroids must be stopped prior to this type of consultation.

Once a diagnosis of allergy is made, the allergist will suggest strategies for preventing and managing your child's allergies. To prevent common perennial allergies to dust and dust mites, the allergist outlines steps for home environmental modifications including the elimination of carpeting, the use of plastic pillow and mattress enclosures, and the use of vacuuming and dusting techniques which avoid precipitating allergic reactions in your child.

What are the recipes for preventing allergies?

Once you identify a trend in your child's nasal reactions that suggests an inhalant or food allergy, the best strategy is to help your child avoid the offending agent or agents. For outdoor allergens, this may mean limiting outdoor play in areas with high concentrations of antigen, such as avoiding play in freshly cut grass. Another maneuver, which will help to prevent allergic reactions, is the frequent use of saline mist nasal irrigations to wash away the allergens and the preemptive use of antihistamines and other anti-allergy medications including leukotriene receptor antagonists, mast cell stabilizers, and corticosteroids. It is often easier to prevent allergies before the fact than to treat them later.

Preventing allergic reactions to indoor allergens, those around the home, often proves difficult. Many of the common culprits may be eliminated or sidelined using strategies I have tabulated for you below.

Table:
Strategies for eliminating environmental allergens

Strategy	Rationale	Detail
Eliminate carpets and upholstered furniture	• Porous surfaces provide hiding places for dust mites, dust, and other inhaled allergens.	• Use wood, linoleum, or tile floors. • Use wooden, leather, or vinyl children's furniture. • Use non-porous slipcovers on upholstered furniture. • Use low pile throw rugs, which are readily washable.
Eliminate clutter	• Porous surfaces provide hiding places for dust mites, dust, and other inhaled allergens.	• Store items, particularly clothes, in drawers, closets, display cabinets with doors.
Allergen-proof bedding	• Porous surfaces provide hiding places for dust mites, dust, and other inhaled allergens.	• Use certified allergen-proof plastic covers for mattresses, box springs, pillows. • Use washable non-wool blankets; use a washable, smooth surfaced bedspread and avoid chenille. • Pillows should be synthetic since foam rubber or feather materials harbor dust mites and mold.

Allergen-proof window treatments	• Porous surfaces and slat, Venetian blinds provide wonderful hiding places and resting surfaces for dust mites, dust, other inhaled allergens.	• Use non-porous, plastic roll up window shades or washable cotton roll blinds. • Avoid slat-type Venetian or mini-blinds, avoid pleated blinds. • May use washable cotton or fiberglass curtains but not draperies.
Use air conditioning and filtering	• Dehumidification and filtration of air is desirable to minimize dust mite, mold growth and to eliminate airborne allergens.	• Central air-conditioners preferable to the dust-scattering air blasting of window units. • Consider use of air cleaner and frequently change air filters
Use controlled humidification	• High humidity favors growth of dust mites and molds.	• Use warm mist humidifier with humidistat and set using humidity gauge.
Toys	• Solid surfaces are safer than porous surfaces; protect toys with porous surfaces from contamination.	• Purchase stuffed toys with vinyl or leather surfaces, washable non-fuzzy cotton surfaces and washable stuffing.
Room decorations	• Avoid dust collectors	• Select furnishings, which have flat, non-ornate surfaces to avoid dust collection. • Do not use hanging mobiles

What are the recipes for preventing allergies?

Preventing allergy symptoms relies upon preventing the chemical mediators which produce them from acting. Agents belonging to 2 major families mediate allergies in the head and neck: the *histamines* and the *leukotriene receptor agonists*. These mediators are released into the tissues when an allergen contacts cells with sensitized receptors. Blocking the action of histamines and leukotriene receptor antagonists, either individually or together, will significantly reduce the frequency and intensity of allergic reactions.

As with all my recipes, you must determine which of these agents used singly or together is most effective for your child. Do experiment with the confidence of knowing that the ingredients may be used together with safety. In general, the ingredients should be started before exposure to allergens both seasonally and episodically. By that I mean that these maneuvers and medications should be used regularly beginning several weeks before the beginning of the spring or fall allergy seasons in order to build up adequate levels of the drug prior to appearance of the antigen. For presumptive spring allergies, begin the medical regimen on April 1st. For late summer and fall allergies, begin the routine on August 1st. Episodic administration of oral or topical agents should begin at least one hour before exposure to the allergens. For up-to-date information about the concentration of allergens in your local air, consult weather websites such as www.weather.com.

Table:
Recipe for preventing nasal allergies

Agent	Mode of Action/ Frequency of Administration	Products
Saline mist nasal irrigation	• Physical elimination and dilution of allergens.	• Simply Saline, Ocean, Little Noses, NeilMed, generic versions, all aerosols.
Keep the home and bedroom allergen-free	• Remove outdoor clothes in the mudroom, wear robe to shower and wash hair	• Air cleaners including HEPA air filters.
Oral antihistamines	• Block binding of histamine to cell receptors.	• *Non-sedating - oral*: Claritin, Zyrtec, Allegra, generics. • *Sedating – oral:* Benadryl.
Topical antihistamine	• Block binding of histamine to cell receptors of the nasal and sinus linings.	• Patanase, Astelin.
Leukotriene receptor antagonist	• Block binding of leukotrienes to cell receptors.	• Singulair
Mast cell stabilizer	• Prevent mast cell release of histamines, leukotrienes.	• Nasalcrom
Topical corticosteroids	• Stabilize cell membranes and inhibit allergic reactions at multiple points.	• Flonase, Nasonex, Veramyst.
Oral corticosteroids	• Stabilize cell membranes and inhibit allergic reactions at multiple points.	• Orapred liquid (prednisolone), oral prednisone.

What are the recipes for treating allergies?

When nasal congestion occurs, particularly if symptoms are persistent and unrelenting compared with the typical acute but relatively short-lived nasal symptoms associated with "colds," allergic rhinitis is likely. Treatment requires a collection of medications, some over-the-counter and some available by prescription only. As is the case with most of my recipes, my regimen for treatment for allergic rhinitis is a step program. Ingredients are added only when additional control of symptoms is necessary. All ingredients may be used together safely and work synergistically.

The recipe for treatment of allergic rhinitis begins with systemic and topical agents directed against the either the histamine and leukotriene pathways of allergy mediation. Studies have shown that these agents that independently block each of the pathways work well together. If the antihistamines and leukotriene receptor antagonist, either independently or together, are less than completely effective, I often suggest the intermittent or continuing use of either systemic or topical decongestants as helper medications. The strongest anti-allergy medications are topical and systemic corticosteroids.

Table:
Recipe for treatment of allergic rhinitis

Step	Rationale	Use	Ingredient/ Measure
Saline mist nasal irrigation	• Moisturization of linings and mucus, cleansing away allergens, contaminants, and diluting mucus.	• 2 sprays in each nostril 3 times a day or more.	• Simply Saline, Ocean, Little Noses, or NeilMed aerosol saline.
Oral Antihistamines	• Blockage of one allergy pathway: histamine-mediated vasodilatation and tissue edema.	• Non-sedating agents used daily.	• Non-sedating: Claritin, Zyrtec, Allegra.
PLUS OPTIONAL Oral Decongestants	• Acute shrinkage and drying of nasal linings.	• Short acting agents in liquid form used up to four times a day for infants and children. • Short acting agents in pill form used up to four times a day for older children. • Extended release versions used every 12 hours for adolescents and adults.	• *Infants*: Sudafed. • *Children*: Sudafed. • *Older children and adolescents*: extended release Sudafed.

Topical Antihistamine	• Tissue blockage of one allergy pathway: histamine-mediated vasodilatation and tissue edema.	• Twice a day.	• Patanase, Astelin.
Leukotriene receptor antagonist	• Blockage of one allergy pathway: leukotriene-mediated vasodilatation and tissue edema.	• Once a day.	• Singulair
Topical cromolyn sodium	• Longer-term shrinkage and drying have swollen and chronically infected or inflamed nasal linings.	• Three to four times a day.	• Nasalcrom.
Topical corticosteroids	• Powerful long-term shrinkage and drying have swollen and chronically infected or inflamed nasal linings.	• Once to twice a day.	• *Infants and young children:* Nasonex.. • *Older children and adolescents*: Flonase, Veramyst..

Topical Decongestants	• Powerful acute shrinkage and drying of nasal linings, often prior to administration of topical nasal steroids.	• **Short acting agents:** 3 to 4 doses/day. • **Long acting agent:** two to three times a day. *Notes*: Use saline mist nasal irrigation prior to a medicated nasal spray.	• *Infants:* **Short acting:** Little Noses Decongestant Drops (1/8% phenylephrine.) • *Older infants and children*: **Short acting:** Mild Neo-Synephrine Nasal Spray (1/4% phenylephrine). • *Older children and adolescents*: **Longer acting:** Afrin (0.05% oxymetazoline).
Antibiotics	• Elimination of bacterial overgrowth due to allergy-driven tissue swelling and mucus production.	• Administration of "rescue" course of moderate, stronger, or strongest class antibiotic.	• Broad-spectrum beta lactamase resistant such as Augmenting, cefdinir.

Meet Lawson

To illustrate the use of this recipe, meet Lawson, an 8 year old with a history of spring seasonal allergies. Since his allergic reactions occur annually with clockwork regularity, he has never had a formal allergy evaluation. He visited me for the first time in early March, the impetus for the visit being his parents concerns that they have been unable to completely control his allergy symptoms.

Mom, dad, Lawson, and I discussed his history. He develops nasal congestion when playing outdoors, and this reaction is usually first noticeable at the time of his birthday on May 5th. He experiences sneezing and nasal congestion spells on the ball field, congestion and cough at night. In the past, his pediatrician has treated his cough with albuterol, a bronchodilator, as Lawson does wheeze from time to time during May and June, especially if he is experiencing one of his frequent spring "colds."

At his first visit, I was not surprised to find that Lawson had a completely normal examination. His nasal linings were not swollen or inflamed. His tympanic membranes and eustachian tube functions were normal. It was March 20, a little less than a month away from beginning of the spring allergy season.

After the examination, we all sat down to formulate a program to start at the beginning of April, two weeks prior to the expected onset of the spring allergy season. I recommended that his folks stock up on all items, both over-the-counter medications and prescription medications, which would be the ingredients in his recipe.

I suggested that he begin the use of saline mist nasal irrigation using the aerosol *Simply Saline* or a store brand on a regular basis as of April 1st. I direct him to use the saline spray three times a day but add additional administrations while he was playing soccer. I suggested that he spray every time he comes off the field. That includes time outs, half time, and whenever he is taken out of the game. For him, it's a nuisance, but so too is sneezing while setting up a critical kick. He complies. I also instruct him to keep allergens from the field out of his home and room. I tell him to shed his soccer uniform in the mudroom or breezeway before entering his house, and I recommend that he take a shower after each game and after each day at school when he has been playing outdoors during gym or recess.

I also suggest that he begin the use of the over-the-counter non-sedating antihistamine *Claritin* on April 1st. Mom buys that drug as a chain pharmacy house brand equivalent. He uses it daily. I also prescribe a canister of *Flonase* for later use. I request that his folks pick up a bottle of the topical nasal decongestant, Afrin, also for later use.

The allergy season begins by the third week of April, but Lawson remains comfortable. His mom then calls me on May 1st with concerns that his symptoms may be outstripping his medications. At my instruction, when his nasal congestion begins to ramp up even though he is using saline and the generic *Claritin*, mom tells him to use *Flonase* once a day. He begins to do so, but, after several weeks, he is having nosebleeds.

Lawson returns to see me, and I note crusting of his nasal linings at the front part of his nose. I tell him to stop the *Flonase* and I recommend local treatment with an extra spray of saline mist followed by over-the-counter antibiotic ointment *Neosporin* or the generic equivalent to each nostril twice a day. In place of the *Flonase*, I prescribe the leukotriene receptor antagonist *Singulair* in an effort to block the alternative allergy pathway that antihistamines miss.

The *Claritin-Singulair combo* works well, and, for the first time in 3 years, he has birthday party during which he blows out the candles on cue rather than with an ill-timed sneeze. By late May, though, he is again fighting congestion, and I recommend that he add back the topical nasal steroid *Flonase*. To prevent any nose bleeding, I suggest that he apply the antibiotic ointment in his nostril after the saline mist but prior to using the steroid in order to protect the sensitive linings in the front portion of his nose. He uses the ointment and avoids nosebleeds.

Mom calls to tell me that she does not think that the *Flonase* is working. She feels that it is not getting into his nasal cavities. I tell her to pull out the *Afrin* and to use it following saline but before the *Flonase*. I suggest that she allow 10 minutes to elapse after spraying in the Afrin before spraying in the topical steroid.

This plans works beautifully for Lawson. In order to minimize his use of the topical nasal steroids, I suggest that he attempt to stop their regular use by mid-June. By that time, the pollen counts have declined and his reactions are well suppressed by the *Claritin-Singulair combo*.

Lawson returns after the July 4th holiday for a checkup. Although he is now off all medications except saline, his nasal linings look perfect. Fortunately, he does not experience allergy symptoms in the fall or at other times of the year. I arrange for him to see me again in March of the following year in order to map the strategy for the next spring allergy season.

9 – About Surgery

What types of surgery help middle ear problems?
What is "tube" surgery?

   When should you consider this surgery for your child?
   What are the benefits of this surgery?
   What are the potential complication and risks of this surgery?
   What follow up is necessary after this surgery?
   Will my child require more than one set of "tubes?"
   What are the details about the operative procedure to insert "tubes?"

What is "adenoid" surgery?

   When should you consider this surgery for your child?
   What are the benefits of this surgery?
   What are the risks of this surgery?
   What are the details of this surgery?

All of the preceding chapters are dedicated to the goal that you will never be forced to read this chapter. That aside, good fortune favors the prepared mind, and learning all that you can about surgery for treatment and prevention of ear infections, middle ear effusions, eustachian tube dysfunction, and hearing loss is time well spent. You will benefit from understanding the risks and benefits of such surgery.

What types of surgery help middle ear problems?

When middle ear infections, middle ear fluid collections, and severe or consistent eustachian tube dysfunction fail to respond to maximal medical management, it is time to consider surgical strategies. Two surgical procedures are available to treat middle ear problems. They are the insertion of "tubes" and the removal of a child's adenoids.

What is "tube" surgery?

The most common surgery for preventing and treating middle ear disease involves the creation of a tiny incision, a **myringotomy**, in the eardrum followed by the insertion of a very small drain called a **tympanostomy tube**. For safety and precision, this operation is performed using a high power stereoscopic microscope while your child is sleeping for a brief time under general anesthesia.

Through the myringotomy slit, we as surgeons vacuum out fluid collections within the middle ear space. Later, any fluid in the middle ear or mastoid cavity that either remains following the surgery or begins to form during an upper respiratory infection will leak out spontaneously. The myringotomy is not only a drain site but also a ventilation port since it permits air from the ear canal to freely enter the middle ear space. This free entry of air then prevents negative pressure with poor eardrum motion, the reformation of middle ear fluid, and the redevelopment of middle ear infection.

Since it requires weeks to months for a child's middle ear disease and the tissue changes associated with it to resolve, we insert an artificial device into the eardrum to hold the incision open. The device is given a variety of names such as the **tympanostomy tube, the ventilation tube**, and **the pressure equalizing or PE tube**. After we insert the tube, we place antibiotic drops into the ear canal to prevent tube blockage or middle ear infection following the procedure.

The tubes themselves are small, about the size and shape of a capital letter "O" on this page. There are many commercially-made tubes available for use. Tubes vary in size, shape, and material. Each is ideal for particular clinical situations. All tubes are constructed of materials well tolerated by the body such as non-reactive plastics, silicone, stainless steel, and titanium. The choice of tube is dictated by the surgeon's preference as well as by the child's clinical situation. Most tubes are held in place by the cut edges of the eardrum. Some tubes, such as the t-tube shown below, actually sit on tiny legs in the middle ear space.

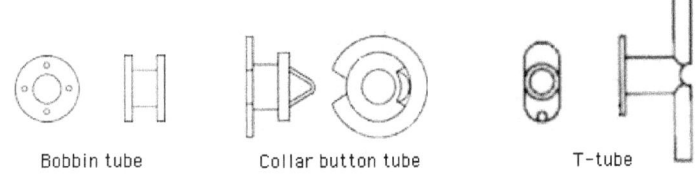

Bobbin tube   Collar button tube   T-tube

Tubes, when properly positioned, will not protrude from the ear canal nor will they fall through the incision into the middle ear. They normally will not be visible except with a special examining instrument, the *otoscope*. How long the tube remains in your child's eardrum depends on many factors including the thickness of the eardrum, the position of the tube placement, and the rate of eardrum growth during the time that the tube is in place. Most small tubes of the bobbin or collar button variety usually remain in place in the eardrum for an average of 12 months. However, the tubes may fall out immediately after insertion or remain in place for over two years. Some tubes, such as the t-tubes, are designed to remain in place until removed by the surgeon. This may be done for an older child in the office without another general anesthesia.

What drives the tube to fall out of the eardrum? The tube seems to be pulled out of the eardrum by the slow growth of the eardrum skin. Eardrum skin naturally migrates as it grows and moves slowly from the center of the eardrum out into the ear canal. The skin tends to carry the tube along with it as it moves. Other forces may precipitate the extrusion of tubes. The tubes may plug with wax or crusts, particularly those that may form if an ear infection occurs while the tube is in place. When plugging occurs, the eardrum may stretch inward and close behind the plugged tube, forcing it out of the eardrum. Because the forces generated by the growing eardrum tend to pull the tube outward, they neutralize any tendency for the tube to fall into the middle ear.

Once the tube leaves the eardrum, the myringotomy incision closes within several days to weeks or even months, depending upon how long the tube was in place. The tube itself may remain within the ear canal for months. Tubes often fall out of the ear canal by themselves or may be removed from the canal as part of an accumulation of earwax. Tubes are usually painless while in the eardrum or after they have fallen out into the ear canal. The only way you will know that the tube is in place is that your child will hear better and will likely have fewer ear infections.

When should you consider "tube" surgery for your child?

The decision to proceed with tympanostomy tube insertion surgery should always be based on a benefit – risk analysis. The benefits are greatest in children who are responding poorly to maximal medical management and whose repeated ear infections and hearing issue create the most significant problems. The following indicators suggest that a child could benefit:

• Persisting otitis media not responsive to combination therapy using the stronger or strongest classes of antibiotics coupled with oral corticosteroids, especially if the child is very irritable, wakeful, feverish and clearly ill;
• Breakthrough otitis media episodes in a child using continuous antibiotic prophylaxis;
• Breakthrough otitis media episodes in a child using episodic antibiotic prophylaxis;
• Repeated spontaneous development of otitis media episodes without accompanying "colds" or upper respiratory infections making it impossible to time antibiotic prophylaxis;
• Repeated development of otitis media associated with eardrum perforations;

• Fluid observed consistently in one or both ears for more than 6 months, even if your child seems to be hearing appropriately and hearing is normal on formal testing;
• Fluid observed in both ears for more than 3 months if your child seems to be experiencing hearing, speech, learning, attention, or behavior difficulties;
• Consistent or fluctuating eustachian tube dysfunction for more than 6 months if your child is experiencing hearing, speech, learning, attention, or behavior difficulties;
• Deterioration of eardrum structure including development of retraction pockets, very saggy eardrum tissue, the beginning of skin debris retention on the eardrum, or the appearance of bony erosions involving the visible ossicles.

What are the benefits of "tube" surgery?

Tubes maintain consistent ventilation of a child's middle ear and mastoid air spaces. They drain fluid that is present as the result of infection and they prevent the reaccumulation of fluid. As a result:

• Ears are less susceptible to the development of middle ear infections;
• Repeated episodic and continuous antibiotic therapy might be stopped;
• Hearing remains consistent and consistently better;
• Ear pain associated with pressure changes in the middle ears is eliminated;
• A child's balance remains consistent and consistently better.

What are the potential complications and risks of "tube" surgery?

A number of undesirable results directly associated with the surgery may occur during or immediately following a myringotomy with tube insertion including:

- Complications of general anesthesia;
- Bleeding;
- Acute ear infections;
- Excessive pain.

Complications may be associated with the general anesthesia administered to your child during the tube insertion. These could include nausea and vomiting with choking, airway spasm called *laryngospasm*, excessive airway swelling, a reaction to one or more of the anesthesia agents, and heart rhythm problems. Anesthetic complications vary from region to region and may also vary with the general health of your child.

Although published studies predict that anesthetic complications could occur in one of every thousand cases, I have not seen a life-threatening complication occur in any of my patients undergoing this type of surgery. Over my 35-plus years of specialty practice, I have never had to admit a child to the hospital for treatment of a complication related to insertion of tympanostomy tubes or the anesthesia for the surgery.

Acute middle ear infections or bleeding may immediately follow tube insertions. I minimize the probability of infection by prescribing perioperative oral and topical antibiotics, the latter in the form of eardrops. Post-operative bleeding around the tube is an event that may lead to plugging of the tube and the need to return to the operating room to clean or to replace it. Bleeding occurs due to excessive eardrum inflammation or unforeseen, minor problems with a child's blood clotting capability. To avoid these issues, I avoid operating on ears with acute or chronic inflammation, preferring to "cool" the ear down first with antibiotic and steroid therapy. I recommend that children having ear surgery also avoid the use of ibuprofen, an agent that interferes with platelet function and clot formation. I suggest that a child avoid *Motrin* or *Advil*, the most common brands of ibuprofen, for several weeks before and after surgery.

Another common cause of post-operative bleeding is a scratch to the ear canal from a child's probing finger. For this reason, I instruct parents of infants, toddlers, and younger children to cut their children's fingernails short before the procedure.

Ear pain following tympanostomy tube insertion is unpredictable. It depends upon the integrity of the eardrum, the level of eardrum inflammation, the amount of surgical manipulation necessary to install the tube, and the child's pain threshold. In general, the discomfort associated with tympanostomy tube insertion may be managed using non-narcotic over-the-counter painkillers, but therapy, as always, must be individualized.

Complications that may occur after the immediate perioperative period include:
• Periodic infections with drainage through the tube due to contaminants entering the middle ear space through the tube;
• An *increase* in the numbers of infections with "colds" and other upper respiratory infections due to the elimination of the natural air cushion;
• Crusting and bleeding around the tube;
• Persistent eardrum perforations;
• Eardrum scarring;
• Eardrum retraction pocket or cholesteatoma formation at the site where the tube rested in the eardrum;
• Requirement for reinsertion of another set of tympanostomy tubes;
• Tube intrusion into middle ear space.

Although the insertion of tympanostomy tubes typically reduces the numbers and severity of ear infections, infections may continue to occur in a percentage of children. That percentage varies with age, and is more common in the youngest infants and toddlers.
These post-tympanostomy tube infections may be driven by organisms entering the normally sterile middle ear space either from the external canal coming in through the eardrum via the tympanostomy tube itself or from the nose and throat coming up

the eustachian tube.

If water enters the ear canal, it may carry bacteria from the ear canal into the middle ear space through the open tympanostomy tube and trigger a localized canal ear infection that then enters into the middle ear space through the tube. A similar middle ear infection and a secondary outer ear infection may be caused in a more conventional fashion if an organism ascends the eustachian tube from the nose and upper throat during a "cold" or other upper respiratory infection and takes hold. This complication is more common in children with poorly managed "colds," and I emphasize to parents that tubes do not eliminate the necessity for managing "colds" effectively. When they do occur, such infections are readily treated and often resolve with the use of topical antibiotics alone. At time, infection resolution requires the combination of topical antibiotics in eardrops and systemic antibiotics administered by mouth.

In a very small group of our youngest patients, the tendency for the child to develop a middle ear infection with "colds" or other upper respiratory infections actually *increases*. This phenomenon may occur due to the elimination by the tube of the middle ear air cushion. Simply stated, the addition of the hole in the eardrum permits the flow of fluid and contaminants up the eustachian tube and into the middle ear space. We all know that it is far easier to pour liquid from a can with two holes rather than a single hole. The tube is that second hole.

When a tube has been in the eardrum or within the ear canal for a prolonged period of time, it may induce a localized infection called *myringitis* with pain, drainage, and sometimes bleeding. Such an infection may be treated with eardrops that contain a combination of antibiotics and corticosteroids.

Persistent eardrum perforations may be avoided by careful follow up and timely removal of tympanostomy tubes that remain in place too long. I will have more to say about lingering tubes in the section to follow.

Scarring and eardrum weakening with the formation of retraction pockets are complications that are usually caused not by the tympanostomy tubes themselves but by the problems that necessitated their placement. Repeated ear infections, middle ear fluid accumulations, and negative middle ear pressures will damage the eardrum's elastic and collagen fibers permitting subsequent negative middle ear pressures to create thin balloon-like pockets in the eardrum. These complications appear more often in children who suffer the recurrence of middle ear disease rapidly following extrusion or removal of their tubes.

For all children who have tubes or who have had tubes, close follow up is necessary. This is particularly for older children and adolescents who tend to be free of symptoms such as pain. Children who have undergone timely tube insertions most often avoid retraction pocket development, even after having the insertion of many sets of tubes. Do not fall into the trap of thinking that your child is on autopilot once tubes are inserted or after they fall out.

In rare instances, particularly in ears which have sustained much eardrum damage, a tube may fall into the middle ear space rather than extrude out into the ear canal. In such cases of *tube intrusion*, a tube remaining behind the eardrum has very little effect on middle ear structures or their function since the prosthesis is constructed of materials well tolerated by the body. The tube in the middle ear space will usually not interfere with a child's hearing. The tube is easily removed through an incision made in the eardrum.

What follow up is necessary after "tube" surgery?

I recommend that an infant or child undergoing tympanostomy tube insertion have careful follow up by the operating surgeon after the surgery. I typically see a child in my office two weeks following the surgery to assess the patency and position of the tubes. At that time, I refer the child for a complete post-operative hearing test, an audiometric evaluation, to be performed 6 weeks to 3 months following the surgery. The delay permits the tube-driven ventilation to return a child's middle ear linings to their normal state prior to testing.

I continue to see the child back in the office at 3 to 6 month intervals, depending upon the child's age and clinical situation. These visits permit me to monitor the position and function of the tube as well as to observe the child for evidence of localized infection around the tube. I also continue to work with the child's parents to managing "colds" and allergies in the interest of preventing ear infections, maintaining hearing at high levels, and avoiding the development of recurring sinus and throat infections.

Tubes should not be left in the eardrums for more than two years to two and one-half years, since the risk of a permanent perforation increases after this period of time. Tubes remaining in the eardrum beyond this time should be removed under general anesthesia in the operating room. When this becomes necessary, I clean the tympanic membrane aperture left by the tube and "freshen" or renovate its edges by disrupting any connections between the outer and inner layers of the eardrum. This maneuver will stimulate the healing process, which then seals the eardrum in the majority of children. Should a perforation occur and persist, it may be patched later with a relatively straightforward surgical procedure.

Will my child require more than one set of "tubes?"

Most children only require a single set of tympanostomy tubes. The insertion of the tube allows air to enter into the middle ear space and permits the middle ear linings to return to a normal state. This may help correct some eustachian tube functional problems relating to blockage at the "ear-end" of the eustachian tube.

The children who experience recurrence of recurrent acute ear infections and recurrent middle ear effusions usually have other issues. Problems occurring at the nasal-end of the eustachian tube, including posterior nasal and adenoidal infections, obstructive adenoids, and muscle malfunctions that impede opening and closing of the eustachian tube, will not be helped by the tube insertion alone.

If middle ear disease does recur in such an instance, I suggest another trial of medical therapy or more extensive surgical therapy, depending on the circumstances of the recurrence. When middle disease recurs immediately after a child's whose previously inserted tympanostomy tubes become non-functional, that child will almost certainly require reinsertion of the tubes and other measures to eliminate throat problems such as adenoidectomy. The time of year and the individual circumstances of the case will ultimately determine the timing and the choice of therapy.

What are the details about the operative procedure to insert "tubes?"

I perform this operation in the operating room at a regional children's hospital. Many surgeons operate in a freestanding ambulatory surgery suite. Parents and the child will usually asked to arrive 60 to 90 minutes prior to the time the operation is scheduled to begin in order to allow sufficient time for necessary pre-operative registration, discussions and examinations.

Prior to the surgery, the parents and the child will meet the anesthetist who will administer the anesthesia. We usually induce anesthesia in the operating room by having a child breathe "laughing gas," nitrous oxide, through a mask. The effect is prolonged and deepened using the safest anesthetic medications in use today, again administered through the same mask. A breathing tube and an intravenous are usually unnecessary due to the short duration of the anesthetic.

Particularly anxious young children may be given a sedative for relaxation prior to entering the operating room. In most operating rooms serving children and their families, one parent or designated family member will be asked to accompany the child into the operating room. A member of the operating room staff will serve as an escort. Once the child has fallen asleep, the parent will be return to the parent waiting room.

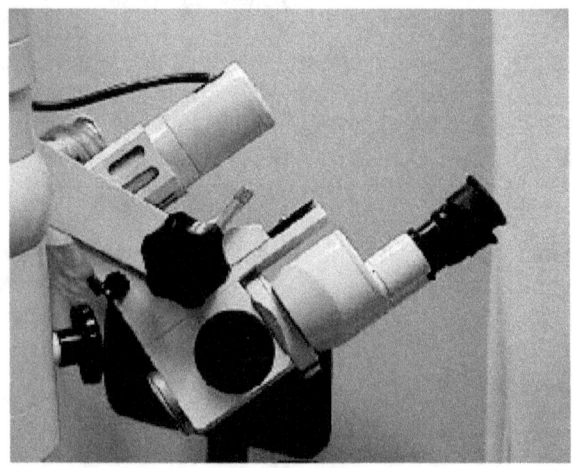

ear surgical microscope

Once the child is asleep, I perform the tube insertion operation using a high power, stereoscopic microscope that magnifies the eardrum and other vital structures within the ear canal. I incise the eardrum with a microscalpel, and I suction out all middle ear fluid. I also observe the status of the middle ear linings as seen through the incision. After the middle ear space is cleared, I insert the tube with microforceps by slowly rotating it into the incision.

After installing the tube, I use it as an irrigation port to wash the middle ear linings repeatedly with sterile saline. If there is any oozing from the cut edges of the eardrum, I instill hemostatic ear drops to cause the microscopic bleed vessels to spasm and clots to form. Following that, I place antibiotic eardrops into the middle ear space through the tube lumen. I also fill the ear canal with the same drops.

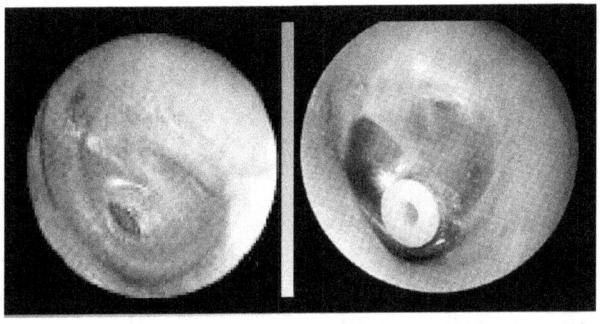

eardrum incision   tube in eardrum

Following completion of the surgery, the anesthetist awakens the child from deep anesthesia and prepares for the trip to the recovery room. At this point, I take the opportunity to speak with parents in the waiting area in order to tell them about the procedure. Your surgeon will likely do the same.
Once the child is settled in the recovery room, parents will be asked to come in to be with her or him during the awakening and recovery process. Be forewarned that most small children are very agitated when they awaken, chiefly due to disorientation from the anesthesia but also due to the sudden appearance of loud sounds and some pain in the ears. This will improve as they awaken more completely, but their agitation will often continue until they leave the hospital, return home, and have a good, long nap.

I give parents instructions to use a higher than routinely recommended dose of Tylenol to use for control of discomfort and pain. I and other surgeons also frequently give parents a security script for a narcotic painkiller such as Tylenol with codeine. As mentioned previously, I recommend avoiding the use of medications such as *Advil*, *Motrin*, or *aspirin* as they interfere with platelet function and may increase the chances of oozing of blood or frank bleeding from the surgical incision as it heals. Even a tiny drop of blood could easily block the tube and create the need for another operation to reopen it.

What is "adenoid" surgery?

Adenoidectomy refers to the surgical removal of the adenoids, a collection of white cell-laden tissues that migrate to the top of the throat at the back of the nose due to repeated nasal or throat infections or due to other stimuli such as allergies. As we have discussed in earlier chapters, adenoidal tissues often enlarge and become acutely or chronically infected as the result of "colds" and other upper respiratory infections. When this occurs, the adenoids may be a source of infection that spreads to the ears, nasal cavities, and the sinuses. Adenoidal tissue swelling at the back of the upper throat may cause eustachian tube functional problems, the development of ear infections and middle ear fluid, obstructive breathing at night as heralded by snoring and breath holding or apnea, sleep disruption, and a reduction in daytime attention and focus.

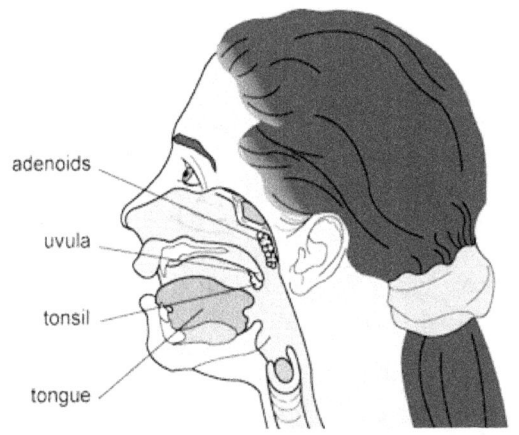

View of Upper Throat Showing Position of Adenoids

When should you consider "adenoid" surgery for your child?

For many years, ear, nose, and throat surgeons noticed that removal of the child's adenoids, either as an isolated procedure or in combination with tonsillectomy, seemed to reduce the incidence of ear infections and the development of middle ear fluid. This observation prompted clinical researchers to perform a series of controlled studies to test the notion that adenoidectomy would statistically reduce ear problems and the need for repeated tympanostomy tube insertions.

In these studies, the test groups consisted of children who had experienced repeated ear problems severe enough to warrant tube surgery not once but twice. With that second operation, the test group also underwent adenoidectomy along with the tympanostomy tube insertion while the control group only underwent tympanostomy tube insertion. When the results were in, the group of children whose adenoids were removed had a significantly lower incidence of subsequent ear infections and fewer of them required a third set of tubes.

Currently, many ear specialists recommend the routine inclusion of adenoidectomy for all children receiving a *second* set of tympanostomy tubes. I personally have no such blanket recommendation, and I feel that the decision for adenoidectomy is influenced not only by the need for a second set of tubes but also by the age of the child, the size and position of the adenoids, the existence of nasal congestion symptoms, the evidence of nasal obstruction, the presence of nasal allergy, and the history of repeat nasal and sinus infections.

Adenoids normally shrink and disappear in older children and adolescents; for this reason, surgery may be unnecessary. On the other hand, adenoidectomy should be considered for a younger child requiring even a first set of tympanostomy tubes if that child is also plagued with recurrent bacterial rhinitis and rhinosinusitis. If a child under the age of 8 or 9 requires a third set of tympanostomy tubes, I recommend that adenoidectomy be included. Large, obstructive, and repeatedly infected adenoids that fail to respond to maximal medical management using my VIP recipes are candidates for surgical removal with or without the insertion of tympanostomy tubes.

Children with cleft palates, either complete and repaired or partial and often invisible to all but the most probing physical examinations, are not candidates for complete adenoidal removal. These children frequently use their adenoidal tissue as a "crutch" to help their palate achieve closure of the tissue valve between the middle and upper throat. Large adenoids also serve as a crutch for those children who have a naturally short palate. If a surgeon removes that crutch, the child may begin to "talk through the nose" and may even experience the back flow of fluids and food up into the nose. This palatal problem can be remedied, but it often requires intense palatal exercises and sometimes reconstructive surgery.

If a child with short soft palate has adenoids that should be removed in order to improve eustachian tube function or airflow through the nasal cavities, a partial adenoidectomy may be performed. Adenoidal tissue may be left in place at the contact point for the palate and otherwise removed from the remainder of the upper throat. Alternatively, adenoidal tissues may be removed only from the sites adjacent to the eustachian tubes.

A frequently asked question is: "If my child is having an adenoidectomy, should the tonsils also be removed?" A number of controlled studies conclude that the routine inclusion of tonsillectomy along with tube insertion and adenoidectomy will not induce a faster or more permanent resolution of middle ear problems. Tonsillar excision may help eliminate middle ear disease if there is evidence that large or chronically infected tonsils are contributing to spread of infection up through the eustachian tube. This may be more common in children experiencing recurring throat infections, streptococcal or otherwise. Since tonsillectomy adds a significant amount of post-operative pain and risk of post-operative bleeding if performed with an adenoidectomy, it should only be included if there is ample evidence that it is necessary.

What are the benefits of "adenoid" surgery?

Adenoid removal removes a potential source of upper throat infection and eliminates a "staging area" for repeated ear infections, recurrent nasal infections, and recurring acute sinus infections. If the adenoids are large and obstructive, their removal will improve a child's breathing and the quality of the voice.

What are the risks of "adenoid" surgery?

Adenoidectomy poses a number of potential risks and may have a number of potential complications. The risks associated with general anesthesia include nausea and vomiting with choking, airway spasm, airway swelling which requires prolonged ventilation with a breathing tube, an allergic reaction to the anesthetics, or cardiac rhythm problems.

Any type of throat surgery may be complicated by the development of post-operative bleeding and infection. Fortunately, bleeding following an adenoidectomy is uncommon, and the amount of blood loss during such episodes is relatively limited. Avoidance of excessive physical activity as well as the use of ibuprofen or aspirin for the first several weeks following surgery will prevent most bouts of bleeding. Infections at the site of the adenoid removal may occur, but they are readily suppressed and eradicated by the use of perioperative antibiotics.

During the surgery itself, despite precautions, the instrumentation used in the performance of the operation may produce complications. The gag used to hold the mouth open must place some pressure on the tongue, lips and teeth. Occasionally, these tissues are unusually sensitive to this pressure. The tongue or lips may swell and become uncomfortable. Teeth, particularly first teeth, may loosen. Should there by a malfunction of the electronic suction device used to cauterize tissues and to seal blood vessels at the operative site, a spark may jump to tissues within other parts of the throat, mouth, or face and create a burn which could cause pain and scarring. This complication is rare but possible.

The longer-term risks of adenoidectomy are upper throat *scarring*, an undesirable *voice change*, and adenoidal *regrowth*. If infection occurs, the raw surfaces left following the removal of the adenoids may scar excessively. This scarring could severely obstruct the back of the nose and require reconstructive surgery.

The voice change risk relates to the development of inadequate palatal closure by the nasopharyngeal inlet valve. The technical name for this problem is *velopharyngeal insufficiency* or *VPI*. I, along with most throat surgeons, carefully examine the palate in the office and again once your child is asleep in the operating room in order to unearth palatal issues before any surgery is performed. If they surface, their complicating effect may be circumvented by the partial removal of the adenoids, leaving residual adenoid tissue in the throat to help the palate effect adequate closure. Rarely, the entire adenoidectomy must be abandoned. Even with these safeguards, unfortunately VPI may periodically occur even though the palate does not appear to be compromised or too short to create an adequate valve.

It is not unusual for adenoidal tissues to regrow, particularly in very young patients or in those patients who have allergies to inhaled materials. Should the adenoidal tissues regrow, they may be removed again. Usually, regrown adenoidal tissue is less abundant than the original adenoidal mass.

What are the details of "adenoid" surgery?

Adenoidectomy is performed on an ambulatory basis under general anesthesia, often along with tympanostomy tube insertion. Since removal of the adenoids is throat surgery, the general anesthesia for this procedure requires the insertion of a breathing or *endotracheal tube* into the upper windpipe to allow safe and painless surgery with the child's mouth open. In contrast, the brief anesthesia for a tube insertion requires only a face mask since it is possible to cover the mouth and nose during this type of brief ear surgery. The passage of the endotracheal tube is a routine part of most general anesthetics, and safety requires the insertion of an intravenous line to allow for the administration of medications during this longer anesthetic.

Surgery is carried out through the mouth without the need for any external incisions. The mouth is held open by a surgical gag, and the tongue is depressed. Before the surgery commences, the soft palate is assessed for length, position, and muscular integrity. If I feel that the palate is currently using some of the adenoidal tissue to help it perform its valvular function in the throat, I may elect to only remove a portion of the adenoidal tissues to prevent loss of effective closure of the upper throat during speaking and swallowing. This will prevent your child from "talking through the nose" or experiencing the reflux of food or fluids into the upper throat or nose.

I remove adenoidal tissue using specially designed instruments that are able to reach up and back into the upper recesses of the throat. Most adenoidal tissue is removed using electronic instruments that electronically vaporize the tissue and then suction away the particles. The same instrument is used to seal open blood vessels and to dry up any residual blood oozing. The adenoidectomy and tympanostomy tube insertion usually requires 40 to 60 minutes to complete.

Following the completion of surgery, the general anesthesia is stopped, the child awakens, and recovery begins in the recovery room. At this juncture, I come into the parent waiting room to review the details of the surgery with parents.

We all, parents and physicians alike, would rather avoid surgery. When it does become necessary, obtain as much detail about the planned surgery as you can from your child's surgeon. Ask questions until you are satisfied with the answers. If you cannot develop rapport with the surgeon, obtain a second opinion and find a surgeon on your wavelength. Once you do, develop a positive attitude and become as comfortable as possible. Your child will readily sense your own reactions and attitudes toward the surgery. If you are tense and nervous, your child will be as well. If you relax, smile, and be positive, your child will follow your lead.

10 -- A Last Word

I end this book as I began it by encouraging you to trust your intuition. You know your infants and children best. Having read the book, you now have the necessary background to prevent and treat ear infections. You also should have the necessary information to frame questions for your child's doctors and to be able to advocate for your child.

When you think about your children, think VIP. Think VENTILATION and INFECTION PREVENTION. As you care for your child, do all that you can do to maintain well-ventilated nasal cavities, throat regions, and, of most importance, middle ear spaces. Integrate measures designed to prevent infections into your child's and into your daily activities. The goal of all my recipes is to help you use common sense and as little medication as possible to maintain your child's good health. I know that you will be able to succeed.

Make checklists for yourself using the information in this book as a template. Use your daily calendar as a memory jog to cue your addition of recipe ingredients and also to track results. Experiment and discover which combinations of ingredients work best for your child and for you. Keep notes, and share both your positive and negative experiences with my program by emailing me at **earinfectioncookbook@gmail.com**. I will be delighted to add your information to this "cookbook" and related publications.

Again, thank you for sharing your time with me. I hope that what I have shared with you has already or will in the future help your child *and YOU* to a happier and healthier life as well as to more restful nights!

11 – *Appendices*

Appendix A: Determining the dose of over-the-counter medications
Appendix B: Determining the dose of over-the-counter medications when no dose is given
Appendix C: Classification of Antibiotics for Treatment of Ear Infections
Appendix D: Dosages of Children's Sudafed Nasal Decongestant

Appendix A: Determining the dose of over-the-counter medications:

Medication	Class	Generic	Recommended dose for age
Claritin	Non-sedating antihistamine	loratidine liquid 5 milligrams per teaspoon loratidine tablets 10 mg per tablet	*2 yrs to 6 yrs:* 1 tsp. ONCE a day *6 yrs and over:* 2 tsp. ONCE a day or 1 tablet per day
Zyrtec	Non-sedating antihistamine	cetirizine liquid 5 milligrams per teaspoon cetirizine chewable tablets 5 mg per tablet	*2-5 yrs, [oral liquid]:* 2.5 mL qd *6-64 yrs. [chewable tablet]:* 5-10 mg qd [oral liquid]: 5-10 mL PO qd
Sudafed Children's Decongestant	Systemic decongestant	Pseudoephedrine	*1 year:* 1 tsp. 4 x a day *6 years:* 2 tsp. 4 x a day *12 years:* 4 tsp. 4 x a day
Little Noses Decongestant Nose Drops	Topical decongestant for infants	Phenylephrine 1/8% nose drops	*Birth to 2 yrs:* 3 drops in each nostril up to 4 x a day, each following saline mist*

Mild Neo-Synephrine Decongestant Nasal Spray	Topical decongestant for younger children	Phenylephrine 1/4% nose drops	*2 yrs to 6 yrs:* 1 to 2 sprays in each nostril up to 4 x a day, each following saline mist*
Afrin Decongestant Nasal Spray	Topical decongestant for older children and adolescents	Oxymetazoline 0.05% nose drops	*6 yrs and over:* 2 sprays in each nostril up to 3 x a day, each following saline mist*

Tsp. = teaspoons
* = Author's recommendations

Appendix B:
Determining the dose of over-the-counter medications when no dose is given:

Most over the counter medications suggest dosages, but many provide no information for children under the age of 6 years and others have no information for parents of children under the age of 2 years. They suggest that you ask your doctor.

When physicians are asked, they usually calculate a safe and effective dose for children under these circumstances by using weight ratios. For example, the *Sudafed* package reads, "For children 2-6 years of age, use 1-2 teaspoons." We begin the calculation, by focusing on the information for a 6 year old. We know that the average 6 year old weighs 48 pounds. Each teaspoon is equal to 5 milliliters. Since the average six year old weighs 48 pounds and should receive 2 teaspoons or 10 milliliters per dose, a 36 pound child would receive 1.5 teaspoons or 7.5 milliliters per dose.   [36/48 x 10 milliliters = 7.5 milliliters or 1.5 teaspoons]

You may use this same calculation method for all over-the-counter medications, assuming that the medication manufacturer provides a recommended dose for a 2 or a 6 year old. The average weight for a 2 year old is 24 pounds, and you may used the same mathematical formula for your calculation.

Appendix C:
Classification of Antibiotics for Treatment of Ear Infections:

Strength Level*	Generic name	Brand Name(s)
Mild	amoxicillin-intermediate strength (70 mg/kg/day)	Amoxil
	trimethoprim-sulfamethoxazole	Bactrim, Septra
	erythromycin-sulfisoxazole	Pediazole
Moderate	amoxicillin – higher dose (80 mg/kg/day)	Amoxil
	cefprozil	Cefzil
Stronger	amoxicillin - clavulanate	Augmentin
	amoxicillin – high dose (90 mg/kg/day)	Amoxil
	cefpodoxime proxetil	Vantin
	cefuroxime axetil	Ceftin
	cefdinir	Omnicef
Strongest	amoxicillin high dose - clavulanate	Augmentin ES
	ciprofloxacin	Cipro
	levofloxacin	Levaquin
	clindamycin – trimethoprim-sulfa	Cleocin – Bactrim or Septra

	ceftriaxone – via injection	Rocephin

* Author's classification

Appendix D:
Dosages of Children's Sudafed Nasal Decongestant:

pounds	milliliters	pounds	milliliters
14	1.3	32	6.7
15	1.6	33	6.9
16	1.9	34	7.1
17	2.2	35	7.4
18	2.5	36	7.6
19	2.9	37	7.8
20	3.4	38	8.0
21	3.8	39	8.2
22	4.3	40	8.4
23	4.6	41	8.6
24	5.0	42	8.8
25	5.3	43	9.0
26	5.5	44	9.2
27	5.7	45	9.5
28	5.9	46	9.7
29	6.1	47	'9.9
30	6.3	48	10.0

pounds	milliliters	pounds	milliliters
31	6.5	49	10.3

About Dr. Smith

Howard G. Smith, M.D. is a pediatric otolaryngologist, a specialist with advanced training and research interests in the ear, nose, and throat problems of infants, children, and adolescents. He is a graduate of Princeton University and the Harvard Medical School with an additional advanced degree in Immunology from Harvard University.

Dr. Smith completed his general surgical training at the Brigham and Women's Hospital and his otolaryngology training at the Massachusetts Eye and Ear Infirmary, both Harvard Medical clinical training programs sited in Boston. Joining the staff of Boston Children's Hospital, he founded the Boston Children's Deafness Network and served as director of otolaryngology at the Eunice Kennedy Shriver Center for the developmentally disabled in Waltham, Massachusetts.

Following recruitment to Southern California, Dr. Smith served as Pediatric Otolaryngologist and Medical Director for the Ross-Loos CIGNA Medical Group in Los Angeles and Orange Counties. He was an attending otolaryngologist at the Children's Hospital of Orange County. Since returning to New England, he has been in private practice at Pediatric Ear, Nose, and Throat Associates in West Hartford, Connecticut, an attending surgeon at the Connecticut Children's Medical Center in Hartford, Connecticut, and a member of the clinical faculty at the University of Connecticut.

Dr. Smith has long been interested in educating the public about health care issues. He is a former medical editor and talk show host at WBZ-AM, WRKO-AM, and WMRE-AM, all in Boston, Massachusetts. He may currently be heard on the podcast "Dr. Howard Smith OnCall" available on Apple's iTunes store and at http://drhowardsmith.libsyn.com/ and many of the subjects discussed in this book are also reviewed.

Education:
- Princeton University, *A.B. in Chemistry and Biology*
- Harvard Medical School, *M.D.*
- Harvard University, School of Arts and Sciences, *A.M. in Immunology*
- National Institutes of Health, Bethesda, MD, *Post-doctoral Fellowship recipient*
- Brigham and Women's Hospital, Harvard Medical School, Boston, MA, *Surgical Internship and Residency*
- National Cancer Institute, National Institutes of Health, Bethesda, MD, *Research and Clinical Associate*
- Massachusetts Eye and Ear Infirmary, Harvard Medical School, Boston, MA, *Otolaryngology Residency*
- American Board of Otolaryngology, *board certification*

Past Clinical Experience:
- Senior staff Otolaryngologist, Boston Children's Hospital, Boston, MA
- Founding Director, Boston Children's Deafness Network, Boston Children's Hospital, Boston, MA
- Associate Surgeon in Otolaryngology, Massachusetts Eye and Ear Infirmary, Boston, MA
- Director, ENT Service at the Eunice Kennedy Shriver Center for the developmentally disabled, Waltham, MA
- Pediatric Otolaryngologist, Ross-Loos CIGNA Medical Group, Los Angeles and Orange Counties, CA
- Attending Otolaryngologist, Children's Hospital of Orange County, Orange, CA

Current Positions:
- Pediatric Otolaryngologist, Pediatric Ear, Nose & Throat Associates, West Hartford, CT, http://www.drhowardsmith.com

- Attending Otolaryngologist, Connecticut Children's Medical Center, Hartford, CT
- Attending Otolaryngologist, St. Francis Hospital and Medical Center, Hartford, CT
- Assistant Clinical Professor, Surgery/Otolaryngology, University of Connecticut School of Medicine, Farmington, CT.

Public Education Positions:
- Former medical editor and talk show host "OnCall with Dr. Howard Smith," WBZ-AM, WRKO-AM, WMRE-AM, all in Boston, MA.
- Producer and host, *Dr. Howard Smith OnCall*, a podcast distributed internationally via iTunes and other aggregators.